Telling the Stories of Life
through
Guided Autobiography Groups

Telling the Stories of Life

through

Guided Autobiography

Groups

James E. Birren

&

Kathryn N. Cochran

THE JOHNS HOPKINS UNIVERSITY PRESS

Baltimore & London

The Johns Hopkins University Press
2715 North Charles Street
Baltimore, Maryland 21218-4363
www.press.jhu.edu

Library of Congress Cataloging-in-Publication Data

Birren, James E.
  Telling the stories of life through guided autobiography groups / James E. Birren and
Kathryn N. Cochran
    p. cm.
Includes bibliographical references and index.
    ISBN 0-8018-6633-2 (hardcover : acid-free paper) — ISBN 0-8018-6634-0 (pbk. :
acid-free paper)
    1. Autobiography—Therapeutic use. 2. Aged—Rehabilitation. 3. Self-help groups.
I. Cochran, Kathryn N. II. Title.
  RC953.8.R43 B575 2001
  615.8′515—dc21   00-011277

A catalog record for this book is available from the British Library.

Contents

Appendixes

Preface

The purpose of this book is to assist people who want to organize and conduct autobiography groups. It provides suggestions on a wide range of issues confronting organizers when developing a program for a group of adults who want to record and share their life histories.

For beginning autobiographers, participating in a group has many advantages over writing in isolation. The group offers a structure that stimulates the recall of events, feelings, and details of settings that might be overlooked or forgotten by an individual writing alone. Also, a lifetime is so rich in details that one has trouble knowing where to begin. A life history can easily become a superficial chronology that misses the important details that define the author's life and personal development.

This manual presents a method of helping people organize their life histories through a *guided autobiography group*. Over the past twenty-five years, this method has proven effective for helping people remember events and experiences from their lives, organize and record them, and share them with others. Guided autobiography offers group participants a starting point; short, structured assignments; the opportunity to discover depth and meaning in life stories through exploration of a variety of life themes; and, most important, the motivation and encouragement of an interested audience. Participants in guided autobiography groups usually express amazement at the power of sharing stories in a small group. An individual reading a personal story stimulates the recall of associated memories for other group members who are listening. Experts now refer to this process as *memory priming*, the power of cues to remind us of things we once knew but have filed away and seemingly forgotten. Listening to the life stories of others refreshes our own experiences. The spontaneous "Oh, yes! I remember that, too" that we often hear during group sharing is evidence of the group's effect on stimulating memories. For the person who is reading, the act of sharing a personal story often brings insights that were not available through the writing alone.

Guided autobiography workshops are organized around a sequence of themes—topics that are common threads in the fabric of just about anyone's life. Branching points, family history, the role of money, the history of one's life work, health and body, development of sexual identity, ideas about death, spiritual life and values, and changing goals and aspirations are universal themes that cross cultural, economic, racial, and gender barriers. The goal is to exclude no one who is participating in the group and to provide enough openness that each individual may respond to the theme and to the accompanying sensitizing questions within the context of his or her own life. The themes move from fairly neutral territory to more personal topics as group trust and personal comfort with the process increase. Participants remain in complete charge of what they share and should never feel pressured to share more than they want to. The last themes encourage participants to create a bridge between past and future.

The process of guided autobiography often rekindles old interests and sparks optimism about the future, which makes thinking about goals and aspirations a natural conclusion to the guided autobiography experience. Sometimes people ask why we have not included such important themes as parenting, education, and exposure to the arts and culture in our core workshop. The reason is that these topics might exclude some people. The themes we have selected allow space for individuals to write about these topics within the exploration of other themes, such as the history of family or work (which would include hobbies). Appendix C contains guidelines for developing themes for specific groups, and we encourage workshop leaders to adapt the themes in ways that support the interests and goals of the groups they are leading.

Interest in forming an autobiography group may come through the structure of an existing group, such as a book club, adult education class, church group, chapter of the American Association of Retired Persons, veterans' organization, or a career-counseling program. Whatever your source of interest in autobiography, you and other organizers face a common question: how can you help people organize, record, and share their life experiences?

Organization and Contents of the Manual

In this manual you will find a wealth of information for group organizers, including background information explaining what guided autobiography is and what benefits it offers to group participants. It contains information on how to plan, organize, and set up a group; outlines for ten group sessions; and appendixes with exercises, handouts, and suggested adaptations for specific groups.

Part I. Background and Workshop Organization

Chapters 1 and 2 link current public interest in the memoirs of everyday people to the speed of change we face in modern society. Autobiography groups encourage people to take the time to take stock of life and the meaning of events, people, and experiences. The process of writing and sharing life stories in a small group stimulates the recall of memories and gives participants an appreciation for the direction their lives have taken and for the courage and creativity they and others have shown in facing life's challenges.

Chapter 1 introduces guided autobiography as a structure for helping group participants organize their memories around major life themes. A series of questions introduces each theme. The "priming" or "sensitizing" questions stimulate the flow of memories, enabling group participants to write full and satisfying autobiographies. Group leaders pose these questions in a rhetorical sense. Group members do not need to answer them literally but are encouraged to react to them and see what comes to mind. The use of themes and related questions releases people from the constraints of a strict chronology and helps underscore the fact that our lives are composed not of a single thread but rather of a complex matrix of events, relationships, and experiences. For part of each session, the large group breaks into smaller groups so that each participant has an opportunity to read aloud two pages he or she has written on the designated theme during the past week and to receive feedback from other group members. Feedback is supportive, encouraging, and nonjudgmental. Chapter 1 describes the benefits of guided autobiography compared with other approaches to memoir writing and life review.

Chapter 2 describes possible target audiences for guided autobiography and its potential uses as a tool for recording family history, facilitating life transitions, enhancing personal development, fostering a sense of community, contributing to the historical record, and having fun.

Chapters 3, 4, and 5 include the kind of nuts-and-bolts information organizers need to set up and conduct a guided autobiography group or workshop. Chapter 3 describes qualifications for workshop leaders. Chapter 4 moves from planning to the details of group organization. It describes the workshop leader's responsibilities; identifies potential audiences; discusses facilities, scheduling issues, and group size; and suggests goals for the group, individual participants, and leaders. Also in Chapter 4, organizers will find practical suggestions for publicizing a workshop and recruiting participants.

In Chapter 5 we present information on how to manage small-group dynamics. In guided autobiography, much of the magic happens in sharing one's life history with others who are on a similar journey. This chapter helps workshop leaders identify and train small-group facilitators. It suggests ground rules for enhancing trust within the small groups, and it discusses how to handle any painful or emotionally charged memories that arise. Every small-group facilitator is a troubleshooter. We present several scenarios that frequently challenge small groups and suggest ways to resolve these problems.

Part II. Session Plans

The second part of the book contains the session plans, detailed outlines for leading ten two- to three-hour group sessions. Each session plan includes objectives, a list of materials required, including handouts (found in Appendix B), and ideas for introducing the new theme for that week. The second half of Sessions 2 through 10 is devoted to sharing in small groups. The last session plan offers ideas for bringing closure to the guided autobiography workshop and suggestions for participants who want to continue writing and polishing their life histories.

Appendixes and Annotated Reading List

The appendixes provide practical information and materials useful in organizing a guided autobiography program and leading a workshop. In Appendix A we present sample fliers and a press release that can be adapted to announce an autobiography program and recruit participants. Appendix B includes all the handouts required for the group sessions. Appendix C offers information on how to develop new themes for special-interest groups, and Appendix D provides suggestions for adapting the material for one-day or two-day workshops. Shorter workshops can spark interest in guided autobiography and often produce potential enrollees for the customary ten-week, once-a-week series of group sessions that constitutes a full guided autobiography workshop. A reading list describes books on autobiography and reminiscence that leaders and group members may find interesting and helpful. The appendixes and reading list support workshop organizers who wish to follow the ten basic session plans that appeal to most general audiences, as well as organizers who wish to adapt the material for the needs of particular groups.

Use of the Manual

We hope that autobiography workshop organizers and leaders will use the material in this manual to bring the experience of guided autobiography to more people. It can give interested and willing organizers the courage and confidence to start a guided autobiography group. All good group leaders are sensitive to the needs of the group and must bring a measure of creativity and flexibility to each group. We have tried to build flexibility into the manual, and we encourage workshop leaders to review, edit, and shape the material to fit their own styles and the needs and interests of the group participants. Taking time to personalize the activities, the discussions, and even the themes will contribute to the success of the leader and the group. We strongly encourage all group leaders to be sensitive to issues and opportunities that arise in the groups during the course of the workshop and to adapt the program as they work to achieve the main goal—to help people organize, record, and share their life stories.

A Good Time to Begin

This is an ideal time to begin guided autobiography groups. There is great public interest in personal histories. Perhaps this is because the Information Age, with its impressive capacity to create databases, focuses on the rapid processing of statistical information while paying too little attention to the personal stories that illustrate how individuals adapt, learn, cope, and grow from the circumstances of their lives. Recording and sharing our life stories can tell us a great deal about who we are and how we came to be the persons we are. Beyond the potential for personal growth, many people are moved to organize and write their memoirs to leave a legacy for their families or, perhaps, for a local historical society or an organization in which they have played a long-term part. We all have a great deal of experience and information stored away in our brains that can be of value to others, and especially to ourselves.

People who have written and perhaps published their autobiographies often put titles on their books that don't use the word *autobiography*. Autobiography is a neutral word, and authors seek titles with words that have more energy and excitement. We use the neutral word because it contains no judgment or expectation. An autobiography is simply the story of a life, an account of the people, events, and influences that gave shape to a life, written by the person who has lived and experienced that life. We do, however, encourage participants to exercise creativity in selecting titles for their own life stories.

Many guided autobiography participants say they find new meaning in their lives through the process of life review and sharing their personal stories with others. Organizing an autobiography can put the uncertainties of the past and the contradictions, paradoxes, and events of life into perspective. Participants become impressed with all they have lived through, the problems they have survived, and the ways they have been tested by people and events. Former participants often tell us that taking part in a guided autobiography group was one of the most significant experiences of their lives.

People of all ages, from eighteen to ninety, have joined the groups. Usually people forty and older have the greatest interest in writing their autobiographies, but anyone in a period of life transition may find it an absorbing and productive task. Transitions from school to work, displacement from work in downsizing, the empty nest of middle age, and retirement all provoke questions about the past, present, and future. Late-life groups, including people facing terminal illnesses, can find the process of recall or reminiscence a peacemaking integration of life experiences. Groups can be mixed by age, gender, and occupational background to achieve the stimulation of diversity. There are also advantages to homogeneous groups, such as veterans or retirees, which can capitalize on a spirit of camaraderie born of common experiences.

Whatever the nature of your group, guided autobiography is a challenging and provocative invitation to write and share life stories in a way that illuminates the richly woven tapestry of life for leader and participant alike. We live in a time of expanding interest in autobiography and personal history. This book is designed to make the process of recalling and organizing life memories both more efficient and more personal. Your use of this book will encourage more individuals to open the treasuries of their life experiences for themselves, their families, and others to appreciate. We wish you well in this adventure.

WE GRATEFULLY ACKNOWLEDGE the hundreds of participants in guided autobiography from whom we have learned so much and who gave many ideas that are presented in this book. Particular thanks are due to those who have participated in the program as group leaders and who have read the drafts of this book and made constructive comments: Pauline Abbott, Betty Birren, Barry Bortnick, Ronald Erlandson, Linda Grant, Helen Kerschner, Blossom Rosen, Elyse Salend, Diane Schmidt, Matthew Solomon, and Cheryl Svensson. Their efforts and enthusiasm have led to many thoughtful improvements in the program and in this volume.

PART I

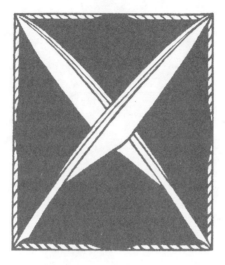

Background and
Workshop Organization

CHAPTER I

The Power of Autobiography

Guided autobiography is a self-enlightening experience. It took me down paths of discovery I had not expected to wander. Coping strategies used over my lifetime unfolded for me so that I could see which ones worked and which didn't. The process allowed me to focus on my potential for success.
—Pauline Abbott

Guided autobiography changed my life. As I relived my life exploring the themes, I relived it through the eyes of an adult. It made me understand things a child could never have understood. All of the sad and unhappy things in my memory bank became just experiences. Knowing more about where I have been helps me know more about where I am and where I want to go. And I get to live the rest of my life one wonderful day at a time.
—Blossom Rosen

What Is Autobiography?

Autobiography is a life history told by the person who lived it, a form of nonfiction writing that dates from the earliest recorded time. Now, at the dawn of the twenty-first century, autobiography is the subject of growing public interest.

Frank McCourt's 1996 Pulitzer Prize–winning memoir, *Angela's Ashes,* fueled an interest in the life stories of ordinary people. The book recounts with humor and sensitivity McCourt's impoverished and painful growing years in Limerick, Ireland. He wrote and published the book after he retired from his career teaching English in New York City.

Readers of McCourt's story realize that they have stories, too. Not everyone's story will have the commercial success of *Angela's Ashes,* but to autobiographers' families and friends, these personal stories will be compelling and treasured.

Autobiography can be a full personal history or a piece of one's history. It can be told in any number of ways. A person may write his or her history as an adventure, profile, humor piece, children's book, or coming-of-age story, or in some other form. Whatever the style, personal histories seem to touch a nerve in both readers and writers. We believe that personal histories are compelling "reads" because they tell us something about who we are and what it means to be human, especially at the befuddling, head-spinning pace of modern life. Keeping up with the whirlwind changes in our high-tech society leaves us little time to ponder the personal details that make up a life.

People need to feel connected to other human beings. Mother Theresa said that Americans are lonely and that loneliness is the most painful form of poverty. Modern life does tend to isolate us. Families are becoming smaller and more fragmented. What family we do have may have followed jobs or dreams to distant places. In two-career households, husbands and wives may work in different cities, seeing each other only on weekends. Not many of us regularly spend weekend afternoons at a family dinner table trading stories with our adult siblings and cousins, aunts and uncles. More of us are running errands we couldn't get done during the week because of work. We rarely settle down to talk about the personal aspects of our lives.

On average, American adults change jobs and residences every five years. Adults entering the workforce today can expect to change careers several times in the course of their working lives. One in three marriages will end in divorce. More adults than ever pass into old age and possible infirmity far away from their children and grandchildren. All these changes can create a sense of isolation from the people and things that could tell us something about who we are. Amid the fast pace and sometimes bruising experiences of life, our uniqueness can get squeezed out like toothpaste from a tube, leaving us feeling empty and discarded.

Writing about our life experiences and sharing them with others gives more meaning to our lives by helping us more fully understand our past and present. The process puts the contradictions, paradoxes, and ambivalence we might find in our past lives into new perspectives. It helps us understand how our personal identity has been shaped by the crosscurrents in our lives.

What Is Guided Autobiography?

There are many ways to describe *autobiography*—life stories, life review, reminiscences, memories, memoirs, and more. The word *guided* refers to preparing a personal history with the help of a tested plan that uses a series of life themes. The themes help us gain access to memories and to organize them in a way that honors the complex threads that shape our lives so that we can present them as a unique and richly woven fabric of life—which indeed they are.

Guided autobiography is a semistructured process for life review that incorporates individual and group experiences with autobiographical writing. In a nutshell, here is how the guided autobiography method developed by James E. Birren works.

Workshop Structure

A guided autobiography workshop is normally presented as a ten-week course, with each weekly session taking two to three hours. The themes may be changed or adapted to meet the needs of specific groups, and the format of the course can be abridged and adapted for one-day or weekend workshops.

Large-Group Work

At the beginning of each session, the workshop leader meets with the entire group of participants for general discussion. At this time, the leader gives participants time to ask questions and discuss problems or insights that came up in the process of writing during the past week. In the large-group session, the leader also introduces concepts related to self-awareness and human development and stimulates the thinking of participants through short writing exercises, paired sharing, and group discussions. At each session, the leader introduces a new theme. Nine themes are suggested in this manual:

1. The major branching points in your life
2. Your family
3. The role of money in your life
4. Your major life work or career
5. Your health and body
6. Your sexual identity
7. Your experiences with and ideas about death
8. Your spiritual life and values
9. Your goals and aspirations

The leader introduces each new theme with priming or sensitizing questions designed to assist in the recall of memories related to that theme. The questions encourage participants to think about aspects of their histories they have overlooked. Through this structure, group members often generate new perspectives on major issues of their lives.

Individual Work

Before each session, individual participants take their own time for personal reflection on the life theme presented. Using the sensitizing questions to stimulate thinking, but with no obligation to answer all or any of them, the individual writes two typed pages of personal history related to the theme. Participants may write more but should select only two pages to read in the small group at the next session.

Small-Group Work

During the second part of each session, each participant reads her or his two pages in the small group and receives encouraging, supportive feedback from other participants, who also read their work and receive feedback.

What Are the Benefits of Guided Autobiography over Other Methods?

Here is a good story for a leader to share with workshop participants. It illustrates the primary benefit of guided autobiography.

There once was an old fisherman who always brought in a full load of fish, even when others with better bait and better equipment came home empty-handed.
"Why is this?" the other fishermen asked the old man. "What is your secret?"
He shrugged. "I know where the fish are," he said.

Guided autobiography will point your workshop participants to the good fishing holes where they are likely to find many memories.

The idea of writing has appeal for many people, but most of us find it hard to get started, hard to get down that first line. Structure helps, and guided autobiography provides structure, stimulation, and that first, compassionate audience. For people with an interest in exploring their personal histories, a guide can provide the encouragement to persist and to mine a deeper vein in their store of memories.

Our lives are so rich in details and so varied that we have trouble knowing where to start. Usually, our first instinct is to start at the beginning, building a linear chronology of events that brought us to the present. This approach, however, can result in bare and boring prose. Our wonderful life histories emerge as a superficial listing of loosely associated events.

Guided autobiography helps autobiographers go deeper. The Birren method shows group participants where to throw in their fishing lines to find the prize fish. The themes provide focus for each session, and the writing assignments are like deep pools. The sensitizing questions that accompany each theme guide the line down to where plump fish are sleeping deep in our memories. Participants in autobiography workshops are almost always surprised at the contents of their catch. By writing about what we find and sharing the writing with others in a supportive small group, we give our memories context and meaning. Also, the shared stories remind other group members of additional events, people, and experiences in their own lives.

Usually the process stimulates so many memories that the biggest challenge for participants is to limit their writing to two pages. Although they may write much more than two pages on a given theme, there are at least two good reasons for the discipline of sharing only two pages per session:

1. The two-page limit is essential to ensure enough time for everyone to share and receive feedback from the group.
2. The discipline of editing to two pages forces the writer to think about which details are most essential to telling his or her story. It requires participants to reflect and to select only the information most pertinent to the heart of their story. The result is focus and clarity, both in the writing and in the way the writers think about their lives. We encourage participants to write freely but to limit their reading in the small group.

Workshop participants will discover that life themes overlap and that they may revisit incidents in their lives more than once. This is normal, and it also provides insight and depth of discovery not usually available by other means.

We would like to emphasize that reading one's work aloud and sharing it with others is as much a part of the process as is the writing, because it is in the sharing that we gain the most insight. In this process of writing and sharing, we can reprogram the way we experience incidents in our lives. For example, an eighty-year-old man wrote of a childhood darkened by emotional and physical abuse by his stepfather, who also abused the man's mother.

> One day when I was about nine, to my surprise, Mother called me to say I should get ready to go with her and the rest of the kids to town. She said further that we were leaving Dad for a while. When Dad, Mother, and all but me were in the buggy, I refused to go along. I've never forgotten the ashen expression on Mother's face and her disbelief. Neither have I forgotten Dad's chuckle and grin of victory. I have since felt that at that moment, I committed Mother to a remaining life of Hell on Earth. Of course, who knows what the alternative outcome might have been had I gone along?

Seventy years later, as he remembered the scene, the man still felt the raw sore of the child's fear and sense of guilt. But in the process of writing about it and sharing his work, he could, for the first time, experience the incident as an adult and look at the nine-year-old he had been with an adult's compassion. He realized that he had been afraid and that his mother must have been afraid, too. The experience changed the incident from a memory that recalled a sense of guilt to one that inspired compassion.

Through the process of writing and then sharing aloud with compassionate group members, individual stories become *our* stories. We learn to value both our individuality and our connection with others. And we learn that part of our humanness is our ability to survive. With humor, perseverance, fortitude, courage, ingenuity, and all the other resources we carry deep in ourselves, all of us have survived a great deal. Autobiography helps bring those strengths to the surface and empowers participants to face their futures with increased enthusiasm and confidence.

Autobiography Can Be Therapeutic, but It Is Not Therapy

Guided autobiography is *not* therapy. Its purpose is not to cure or improve psychological, social, or emotional problems. Nevertheless, it often can be therapeutic. Like regular exercise, enjoying a cup of tea in the garden, conversing with a trusted confidant, playing a musical instrument, gardening, or spending leisure time in nature, autobiography has healing powers. It does not have as its specific goal a change in behavior or emotions, but positive changes may result. Changes usually occur through the resolution of longstanding issues or through rediscovery of the passions and interests of the inner child. In addition to the written stories, the principal product of autobiography group work is *insight*. And insight can be achieved by a guided walk through life in the company of others who are on the same journey.

CHAPTER 2

Who Should Do Autobiography?

Our lives that seemed a random and monotonous series of incidents are
something more than that; each of them has a plot.
—Malcolm Cowley

One writes to make a home for one's self, on paper, in time, in others' minds.
—Alfred Kazin

Life *is* story. We experience its twists and turns, its plot points, its rising and falling action. But the plot direction and the cumulative significance of events can become lost to us in the routines of daily living. Our lives may feel routine and monotonous, hardly worth writing about. Yet buried in the details of each individual life is unique autobiographical material that has universal human interest. This is true of people at any age and from any background.

There are countless good reasons to encourage people to write down and share their story or stories. A guided autobiography workshop is particularly appropriate for people who want to

1. leave a legacy for family members;
2. facilitate life transitions;
3. enhance personal growth and development;
4. build a sense of community;
5. contribute to history;
6. enjoy the thrill of self-discovery.

Information in this chapter provides a sound background for workshop leaders. Many of the ideas and examples provided below will be useful for group discussions during the workshops.

Leaving a Legacy for Family Members

A personal history is a moving gift for family members. Grandparents often think of doing this late in life to leave something behind for their children and grandchildren. That is great; but the impetus for sharing personal history needn't wait until ripe old age. Students in a gifted and talented English class at James Madison Memorial High School in Madison, Wisconsin, were asked to list ways in which adults could improve communication with teenagers. Among their top ten recommendations was, "Tell us stories about when you were little and when you were a teenager. The stories don't always have to teach a lesson; they are fun!"

These teenagers are asking to know adults better as fully fleshed-out people. They want to know about adults' feelings and struggles when they were young. They want to know that funny, embarrassing things happen to other people, even adults, and that people recover from them and can laugh about them later. Knowing more about their parents and grandparents or other adults in their lives can help young people know themselves better.

Most of us are intrigued by our roots and would like to know more about our parents and our ancestors because their stories are connected to our own. A middle-aged woman came to a guided autobiography workshop looking for distraction from the challenges of raising teenage children who were questioning values she held dear. The group was working on family histories. This is what she wrote.

When I was five, my family moved from my grandparents' farm to a town about fifty miles away where my father started a small business. Soon after the move, my best friend and brother, who was only eighteen months older than I, became seriously ill. He had to stay home from school and undergo many surgeries. I didn't know it until I was an adult, but the doctors told my parents they didn't expect him to survive a year. He rode the cusp of many medical advances and survived to forty-nine, but his health problems had an impact on our whole family. When he got sick, I was six. I had a three-year-old sister and an infant brother who also was hospitalized several times in his first year. I had to grow up fast to help with chores and help care for my younger siblings. The family values of hard work, caring for others, self-sacrifice, and fiscal conservatism were absorbed by me very early. I think I poured all my own pain and sense of loss into trying to make things easier for my mother. I was praised for my maturity and capabilities, and I think the responsibilities I had did give me a feeling of pride and self-confidence. I wanted to do everything perfectly so that I would not create any more stress for my mother or draw any negative feedback to myself. I didn't want to make any more waves!

Now my kids tell me I am too perfectionist. They complain that I am overly critical, always looking for what is wrong or unfinished. As I write this, I am remembering an apron my mother has that my great-grandmother mended nearly one hundred years ago. The pattern is so perfectly matched and the hand stitches so tiny and flat that the mend is barely visible. And this on a kitchen apron used on the farm! I guess perfectionism has a long history in my family. These are some of the sayings I grew up with:

"A job half-done isn't really done at all."

"If something is worth doing, it is worth doing right."

"If you raise the first child right, all the others will follow."

It drives me nuts when my kids whine at doing chores or do them only halfway. It makes me wonder if I have been a good parent. So I try harder! I think the kids are asking me to lighten up and chill out a bit. Maybe that isn't a bad idea after all these years. I wonder if anyone ever asked my great-grandmother to lighten up.

Most families groan at the superficial stories that have been told time and again or that have leaden, overworked morals. The stories we really want to hear reveal to us through the events and details of life something about the characters of the storytellers and their worlds. We want to know what went into the choices they made, what things mattered to them, how they learned, and what they really wanted from life. Few of us talk about things of this depth at family reunions. And we don't all have family reunions. In this land of immigrants and movers, many children do not know their grandparents. Some of us have no family with whom to share our history, but every one of us belongs to the larger family of humanity. Participants in a guided autobiography workshop have the opportunity to find a sense of family in their small groups and to share something of their histories with others. The legacy and impact of a personal history are not limited to bloodlines.

Facilitating Life Transitions

In 1831, French historian Alexis de Tocqueville wrote of Americans, who so fascinated him:

> Born often under another sky, placed in the middle of an always moving scene, himself driven by the irresistible torrent which draws all about him, the American has no time to tie himself to anything, he grows accustomed only to change, and ends by regarding it as the natural state of man. He feels the need of it, more, he loves it; for the instability, instead of meaning disaster to him, seems to give birth only to miracles all about him.

De Tocqueville captured the American restlessness and passion for progress that drove the westward movement and continue to drive the rapid pace of change in our contemporary society. However, he did not write about the discomfort and confusion individuals usually feel while going through transitions.

In his book *Transitions: Making Sense of Life's Changes*, William Bridges writes, "To be 'up in the air,' as one so often is in times of personal transition, is endurable if it *means something*—if it is part of a movement toward a desired end. But if it is not related to some larger and beneficial pattern, it becomes simply distressing."

Bridges points out that transitions are especially difficult when the things we are leaving or going to also are changing. "Stuck in transition between situations, relationships and identities that are themselves in transition," he writes, "many Americans are caught in a semi-permanent condition of transitionality. It is as if we launched out from a riverside dock to cross to a landing on the opposite shore—only to discover in midstream that the landing was no longer there. (And when we looked back at the other shore, we saw that the dock we left from had just broken loose and was heading downstream.)"

Guided autobiography, with its combination of personal reflection, writing, and sharing of the writing with a supportive group, can help in the difficult process of leaving behind an old situation, making some sense of the awkward and uncomfortable in-between phase, and finding clarity, courage, and enthusiasm for the phase ahead. Autobiography places a transition in the context of a life. With a better understanding of our past, we can move ahead with a sense of continuity, taking some things (such as personality traits, values, a belief system) forward with us and leaving others (a job, a marriage, a former home, a dream) behind with a freeing sense of resolution. And we can meet the new situation with a stronger sense of direction and purpose. In other words, guided autobiography can provide a better sense of the larger life journey of which the current transition is a part. It situates a transition in a larger, beneficial pattern.

Bridges views transition as "the natural process of disorientation and reorientation that marks the turning points of the path toward growth." Some transitions are involuntary and devastating—the loss of a beloved spouse or child, the loss of a job, injury or illness that demands a dramatic change in lifestyle, an unwanted move, forced retirement, financial difficulties. Even joyful, voluntary transitions, such as marriage, the birth of a planned child, a job promotion, or a wanted move, can be difficult. Every transition involves change, the loss of a known situation, and movement into the uncertainty of a new situation. A couple of stories illustrate this.

A woman, after years of hard work, was named the chief executive of her company. The promotion marked the achievement of a long-held goal, but she was strangely sad. She missed the camaraderie she felt with her peers at her previous level of management. Now, she realized, it truly is lonely at the top, but believing her sadness was inappropriate, she hid it. In an autobiography workshop, she aired her feelings in writing about the history of her career. For the first time she recognized that the camaraderie she had felt before might no longer be possible on the job, so she decided to become more involved in volunteer endeavors with other executives in order to develop a new peer group less closely related to her work.

A man in his mid-fifties had a severe heart attack and was advised by his doctor to change his lifestyle to reduce stress. This athletic and energetic man was forced to find new inner strength to cope with the long recovery and his fear of another attack. He struggled to understand what life could be for him with his new physical limitations. In writing his autobiography, he recalled stories about games that he had invented as a child and about the creative ways in which he had motivated the sales force he managed for his company. It occurred to him that the innovative strategies he had used throughout his life could help him adjust creatively to his altered lifestyle. He realized that he had more control over his future well-being than he had thought, and he began to view his transition in a more positive light.

Transitions, like the beat of a drum, add rhythm and texture to life. Each life has not only its own rhythm but also a melody line that moves forward from one phase to the next. The melody line includes those aspects of the self and personal history that we choose to carry forward. These personal assets and our external support systems can provide continuity and help us adapt to new situations.

Kierkegaard said, "Life can only be understood backwards, but it must be lived forwards." Autobiography can serve as a bridge that helps us travel more easily from our past to our future.

Enhancing Personal Growth and Development

Over the past thirty years, formal research conducted by a variety of professionals to assess the impact of life review and autobiography has shown that, in the adults studied, the process of life review provided measurable gains in emotional well-being and practical capabilities. These findings corroborate the positive comments, letters, and evaluations we have received from participants in guided autobiography workshops. People who participate in a life review process, such as guided autobiography, report these results:

- Increased self-esteem and a greater sense of personal power and significance
- Greater awareness of past adaptive strategies and ways in which these might be applied to current problems and conditions
- Resolution of past resentments, pain, and negative feelings and a sense of reconciliation
- Renewed interest in past activities and hobbies
- Ability to differentiate between the roles of enduring internal motivations and external societal motivations in making life choices
- Development of friendships and confidant relationships with other group members

- An increased sense of meaning in life
- Appreciation for the developmental work one faces at each stage of life
- A greater sense of accomplishment and fulfillment
- A stronger, more positive view of the future

Because of these outcomes, guided autobiography can be a useful tool for recovery groups, religious groups, adult education classes, women's groups, men's groups, adolescents' groups, or any other group whose members are interested in an increased awareness and understanding of themselves and their relationships to others. It also may be a useful tool for psychologists, psychiatrists, social workers, and other mental health professionals.

Many things influence the turns we take in life. Finances, health, personality, our parents, our ethnic roots, our personal fears and insecurities, societal values, and luck all play a part. The capacity for individual growth, however, depends on recognizing and taking responsibility for one's own choices. We cannot view our lives as problems caused by others if we want to open the door to personal growth.

Guided autobiography provides an opportunity for the kind of introspection and group sharing that help us examine and leave behind the wounds of childhood, rethink the expectations of parents and society, reassess our own aspirations and goals, and reaffirm personal needs, interests, and ambitions so that we can move on to a more authentic and balanced future.

Inevitably, life review at any age—but particularly for middle-aged and older adults—involves a comparison between life as it has been lived to the present and life as it might have been lived. It offers an opportunity to reconcile past values and goals with present realities. Like cleaning out a closet, guided autobiography is an invitation to make some choices about what to keep and what to throw away.

A man in his mid-fifties had been a successful executive in a major corporation for many years, but lost his job in a hostile takeover. At his age, in an industry confronting consolidation and downsizing, he thought his chances of finding a new job in the industry were slim. He felt desperate and, in his words, "wadded up and thrown away." Through guided autobiography, he remembered how much he had enjoyed working with teenagers when he was a college student and how often he had been a mentor to young managers entering his company. He realized he had always wanted to teach but never thought he could afford to and still live the lifestyle to which he and his wife had become accustomed. But now his children had finished college, and he had invested wisely enough to have a reasonably secure retirement. He decided to pursue teaching math in high school. His wife had been an English teacher and was willing to return to teaching for the additional income it would provide. They looked forward to this second career and the three months of summer vacation each year in which they would be able travel. He felt a sense of freedom and purpose in his pursuits that he had not felt in many years.

Through participation in a guided autobiography workshop, this man was able to find a new value in his past career, not only as a manager but also as a teacher and mentor. The rediscovery of satisfying old interests gave him a stronger sense of himself, and he liked what he saw. The experience reaffirmed the value of his past life and also provided the closure he needed to end his grieving over his lost job and to move on. He could not control the downsizing, but he could control what he did with the challenges and opportunities the period of unemployment presented.

Participation in guided autobiography also gave this man tools for self-exploration, introspection, and building confidant relationships that are likely to help him continue to grow throughout the second half of his life.

Building a Sense of Community

We have already discussed how guided autobiography can help us with transitions. There is another valuable by-product of autobiography that is also very important in our supercharged, rapidly changing, measured-in-megahertz contemporary environment: it builds a sense of community.

Family, neighborhoods, a long career with a single company, and other institutions that once contributed to a sense of stability in our daily lives have suffered in the whirlwind of modern life. Frequent moves, divorce, distance from extended family, jobs that demand long hours or a lot of travel, and a restless personal search for social and economic improvement have become fairly common. So much unrelenting change challenges the development of a sense of community or belonging—anywhere. In the midst of the Information Age and the shrinking world, many people feel isolated.

Guided autobiography emphasizes the importance of sharing our stories with others. At first, participants may feel guarded and reserved, but they soon begin to feel part of a supportive family. They are able to share the dark aspects as well as the lighter episodes of their personal histories. Guided autobiography welcomes the presence of the whole person. All of us have suffered pain and setbacks in our journeys, as well as triumphs and joy. In sharing our stories and hearing those of others, we realize that, while the details of each story are unique, we all have endured and come through pain as stronger people. We are here. We are survivors. Ernest Hemingway said, "The world breaks everyone, and afterward, many are strong at the broken places."

In his book *The Story of Your Life: Writing Your Spiritual Autobiography,* Dan Wakefield writes, "The sharing of experience at the personal level brings us closer together, shows us the commonality of our humanity." One of Wakefield's students, a banker, found the discovery of "the similarities in our [autobiography group members'] lives was a great revelation. The sharing of experiences and hearing others describe theirs was a highlight of every week." We have found that many guided autobiography groups continue to meet and share experiences after the formal workshop has ended, so strong is the participants' sense of commitment to one another and their interest in discovering more about themselves and what it means to be a human being.

The community-building aspect of guided autobiography makes the process particularly useful for building a sense of community in a variety of settings, such as orienting new members to a church, encouraging tolerance in ethnically diverse communities, or fostering new friendships in a retirement home.

Even if the guided autobiography workshop is only for a weekend, participants typically experience a strong sense of community with their colleagues. Stepping out of the rat race gives us time to think and feel. We feel more alive and valued when our thoughts and feelings are shared and honored by others. Hearing other people's stories triggers more of our own memories, often memories that link the experiences of group members. The sharing broadens our perspectives and can lead us to think of our lives in a different way. The autobiography group is a small but vibrant community that provides individuals with support, recognition, and a context in which to better understand the significance of their life experiences. Participants become invested in the well-being of their fellow group members.

Contributing to History

Several years ago, the Smithsonian Institution in Washington, D.C., was putting together an exhibition on the migration of African Americans from the rural South to the industrial centers of the North. The curators wanted to show how life had changed for African Americans as a result of the migration. Researchers interviewed families across the country. People generously shared letters and formal portraits of their ancestors and the stories that had become part of family oral histories. But they could not provide a category of things the curators really wanted for the exhibition—items of daily living. The maid's uniforms, kitchen utensils, farm tools, worn clothing, furniture, and suitcases had been thrown out long ago. These mundane articles represented hard times and were not thought worthy of keeping.

The editor of *Smithsonian* magazine put out a plea to all readers, asking them to think twice before throwing out items that illustrate how we live day to day. Just as the utensils and work uniforms of African Americans gained significance in the context of a historical exhibition, so the mundane details and events of life take on greater significance when they shed light on the plots, themes, and characters in a personal history.

Autobiographies can be useful to historians in the same way that letters and diaries have been useful primary sources for historians in the past. These personal stories reflect how people lived in a particular time, place, or culture. They illustrate how individuals responded to events and to the social, political, and financial currents of their time. They make the personal struggle for survival and happiness real. No amount of statistical information, now so readily available in our computerized databases, can provide that personal perspective.

If we keep all our memories in our heads, if we don't take them out to examine them, give them shape and substance, and record them, they will be lost to our families and to future generations. Much of the narration in Ken Burns's award-winning documentary on the Civil War was drawn from letters—letters from mothers to sons, from soldiers to lovers, from generals to presidents. In an age when a personal letter arriving in the mail is almost as rare as a snowflake on the Sahara, autobiography assumes even greater significance than in the past.

The Thrill of Self-Discovery

Group leaders can help workshop participants uncover the plots and themes of their lives. No matter what the age of the writer, autobiography is a story in progress, a slice of a whole. Autobiography can take the form of a thriller, humor book, mystery, nature story, documentary, romance, children's book, journal, book of poems, or letter. No one other than the writer can say what is right or wrong, true or false. Interpreting a life is the responsibility of the person who lived it. Nobody else has access to the memories or feelings. Participants write their stories as they see them. And, as life flows through them onto the page, they are likely to feel very much alive, challenged, and ultimately capable. They are usually amazed at how much they have to say and how eager they become to say it. Recounting the story of one's life is a valuable experience that should be available to everyone.

CHAPTER 3

Qualifications of the Leader

Certainly, travel is more than the seeing of sights; it is a change that goes on, deep and permanent, in the ideas of living.
—Miriam Beard

The events in our lives happen in a sequence in time, but in their significance to ourselves, they find their own order . . . the continuous thread of revelation.
—Eudora Welty

Guided autobiography is a journey for both workshop leaders and participants. Even though participants are writing about the events of their own lives, their involvement in a guided autobiography workshop can be like taking a journey into the unknown. Surprising memories, feelings, associations, and insights arise. People setting out on an uncharted adventure, such as guided autobiography, naturally seek the help of a qualified guide. That is the role of the workshop leader.

Workshop leaders need to be prepared to encourage participants, help them gain access to their memories through group discussion, and support them when they encounter ambiguities as they write and share their life histories. This should be done without any overtones of judgment or evaluation that might embarrass participants or make them feel reticent about writing or sharing their life stories.

Guided autobiography is not a form of therapy designed to solve problems or heal the sick. Participating in an autobiography group can lead group members to personal insights and experiences that may feel therapeutic to them, *but group leaders should not act as therapists.* Instead, the leader's efforts should be focused on helping participants organize, record, and share the real events of their lives without encouraging a problem-solving atmosphere. Guided autobiography provides opportunities for group members to learn, grow, and discover more about who they are. Their guides need not be licensed therapists or psychologists, but certain qualifications do apply. Leaders of guided autobiography workshops should be

1. alumni of earlier autobiography groups;
2. experienced in teaching or leading small groups;
3. supportive, empathetic, enthusiastic, and kind;
4. well organized and flexible;
5. well-read in autobiographical and other writing;
6. good listeners and communicators;
7. possessed of a good sense of humor;
8. humble;
9. committed and interested.

Previous Participation in an Autobiography Group

Participating in a guided autobiography group is an essential preparation for leading a workshop. The experience of having sought meaning in one's own life and, even more important, having risked sharing one's personal history with others fosters a sensitivity and respect for the process. Leaders who have experience as an autobiography group participant have a better appreciation for how trust builds within the group over time. They understand from personal experience the most helpful kinds of support and feedback other group members and the leader can provide. They have a clear understanding of the process and are familiar with its structure, and they have seen how another leader fielded questions and dealt with the diversity of experience and temperament within a group.

Experience Teaching or Leading Small Groups

A leader is responsible for presenting the themes and related materials, motivating and inspiring participants, and managing the group to maximize the benefits of participation for all group members. This means drawing out shy members, preventing a few from dominating the discussion, keeping the tone of discussion positive and supportive, and troubleshooting problems as they arise. Training in such fields as social work, pastoral care, nursing, psychology, or teaching, especially combined with previous experience leading small-group discussions, is very helpful, but not absolutely essential. Any leader, however, must be sensitive to how individual members and the group as a whole are experiencing the guided autobiography process and must have good problem-solving skills.

Ability to Be Supportive, Empathetic, Enthusiastic, Kind

Participants naturally feel a bit uncertain at first about the process of writing and sharing their life histories. They may be afraid that they are not good writers, that their stories are less interesting than others', or that they will be ridiculed or criticized. It is important to remind group members that the objective of a guided autobiography group is not a polished, finished product but the opportunity to begin imposing some order on a life's wealth of memories, to learn more about oneself, and to find meaning in one's own life story. This is the endeavor for which the group leader provides support. For people who want to complete a polished, finished autobiography, guided autobiography is a reconnaissance trip.

Leaders of autobiography groups must also be sensitive to the unexpected emotions that the recall of distant memories can evoke. The group leader must respect spontaneous expressions of emotion, showing empathy—often just through facial expression or a gesture, such as offering a tissue—while avoiding protracted discussion of the incident or evaluative comments. The leader should strive to develop an atmosphere that incorporates the expression of feelings into the normal flow of activities. To enhance the process of memory retrieval and self-discovery, the leader must be able to establish a tone of tolerance and encouragement, as well as respect for the degree to which individual participants wish to share.

Good Organizational Skills and Flexibility

We live in a busy world. Although participants use an autobiography group as an opportunity to pause and reflect, they also like to know where they are going and why. They want to feel they are using their time wisely. Starting and finishing on time and managing group sessions so that everyone can participate in the discussion and share their work are very important. Leaders must be sure the facilities are ready and adequate, the handouts and other supplemental materials prepared and relevant.

At the same time, the leader should be willing to adapt plans to meet the needs and interests of the group. Evaluating the needs of the group and making appropriate adjustments is a subtle but ongoing process throughout the workshop. Leaders should ask for feedback and questions at the beginning of each session, and should also watch for clues in body language and facial expression. The leader must be knowledgeable and well-prepared enough to move through some material more quickly if the group's interest is low and allow extra time to explore material the group finds more interesting.

Familiarity with Autobiographical and Other Writing

Leaders should be familiar with contemporary literature on autobiography and reminiscence and should be generally well-read and curious. A leader who is both well-read and intuitive can greatly enhance the workshop by bringing in additional information and insights that reinforce the discoveries and insights group participants will have on their own. A story, a writing technique, a quotation, or a newspaper article can add to an individual's understanding of his or her journey and underscore that we are not lone travelers. Learning is part of our human condition, and opportunities for new understanding and perspectives are available from many sources. The leader acts as the heart of the group organism, pumping nourishment and encouragement to individual participants while at the same time attending to the health of the larger group.

Good Listening and Communication Skills

The ability to listen carefully, to provide appropriate, well-articulated feedback, to speak clearly, concisely, and warmly, and to effectively resolve any problems that arise in the group are hallmarks of a good guided autobiography workshop leader.

A Good Sense of Humor

Humor helps release tension and can make difficult memories easier to confront. Many of the life themes explored in guided autobiography generate discussions of sensitive topics among people with quite different points of view. A humorous story or one-liner can reduce tension. Sharing a laugh facilitates bonding and encourages participants to use humor in their writing and in their discussions. Participants will enjoy pursuing their autobiographies in the pleasant, collegial manner that humor fosters. Group leaders should try to have at least one humorous story to tell at each workshop session, a story related to the theme being introduced. There are many books devoted to jokes and humorous quips on such relevant topics as work, family, and health; these are available in most bookstores and libraries.

Humility

The best workshop leaders realize they also are students of life, facilitators not gurus, with strengths and weaknesses of their own. They are aware that they can learn a great deal from the group. In guided autobiography, the leader is not really an expert imparting knowledge to the unlearned. Instead, the leader acts as a guide helping the participants become conscious of knowledge they hold within themselves. The traditional judgments that often apply in education—answers that are right or wrong, actions that are correct or incorrect, better or worse—do not apply. Leaders should approach guided autobiography with a humble respect for the dignity of each individual life journey. Personal agendas should not take precedence over commitment to the growth and well-being of the group and of individual group members.

Commitment and Interest

Being a group leader takes commitment, time, and energy. A sincere interest in people and their stories combined with a desire to use the tools of guided autobiography to help people organize and share their stories—these are essential qualities in a group leader.

CHAPTER 4

Organizing a Guided Autobiography Group

*Life begets life. Energy creates energy. It is by spending oneself
that one becomes rich.*
—Sarah Bernhardt

*The artist must have some kind of order or he will produce a very small
body of work. To create a work of art, great or small, is work,
hard work, and work requires discipline and order.*
—Madeleine L'Engle

———————————

Organizers of autobiography groups set the tone for the success or short-
comings of what amounts to an exploratory expedition into life history. As
with any expedition, a serious guide prepares in advance, motivates and in-
spires members of the expedition during the journey, and evaluates the expedition and its successes and failures at the end. The guided autobiography
leader usually

1. identifies the audience;
2. sets personal goals and group goals and supports participants in setting their individual goals;
3. recruits participants;
4. adapts materials to the needs of the group;
5. schedules the time and location of group sessions and arranges for
   facilities (room, furniture, audiovisual equipment, photocopies, coffee, etc.);

6. guides the group process by preparing and leading group sessions;
7. provides support to group participants and feedback to staff, if the autobiography group is sponsored by an organization.

Sometimes the execution of these responsibilities is shared with the staff of a sponsoring organization, but the workshop leader is ultimately in charge of seeing that the details that enhance the guided autobiography group experience are attended to. (Responsibilities listed in items 6 and 7 are dealt with in detail in Chapter 5.)

Identifying the Audience

Guided autobiography is appropriate for many types of groups. We have led groups at universities and community centers in the United States and abroad that included participants from widely diverse backgrounds—men and women ages twenty to more than ninety of diverse ethnic and socioeconomic backgrounds and diverse career tracks. The variety of perspectives was in itself enriching. Heterogeneous groups may be recruited through local libraries, community adult education programs, community groups, churches, colleges or universities, and counseling centers.

Guided autobiography is appropriate, too, for groups of people with similar experiences and goals. While the participants may have some life experiences in common, they process those experiences in the context of a larger life story that is unique. The sharing of personal life histories will trigger more memories in other participants and broaden the context within which individuals experience both their shared backgrounds and the unique details of their own lives.

The list of possible audiences is endless, but here are a few ideas:

- New members of a church
- Recent retirees
- Veterans of the same war
- Concentration camp survivors
- Executives in outplacement programs
- Recovering substance abusers
- Women seeking re-entry to the workforce

- Young mothers seeking a sense of balance between career and family responsibilities
- Retirement home residents
- Schoolteachers interested in introducing autobiography to their students
- Any group trying to assess the impact of a particular life experience, such as the Great Depression; college in the 1960s; facing cancer or other chronic or life-threatening illness; adjusting to divorce or the loss of a spouse

Setting Goals

Group Goals

The goals for the group will be influenced by the leader's or sponsoring organization's reasons for offering guided autobiography. Here are some examples of group goals determined by the particular nature of a group:

- To help build a sense of community in a new setting, such as a church community, a retirement home, or a support group for new retirees
- To develop strategies for coping with life transitions, such as career change, empty-nest syndrome, loss of a spouse, living with a disability, or adjusting to life after prison
- To help participants understand how they came to be where they are in life and to explore alternative directions for the future
- To find internal resources to face difficulties, such as job loss, impending death, chronic illness, or a loss of any kind

These specific goals may be in addition to the following, more general goals that apply to the members of any guided autobiography group:

- To develop new acquaintances and a sense of community within the group
- To recall, organize and write, and share life stories
- To explore various strategies for coping with the joys and difficulties of life

- To examine issues related to adult development
- To trust and honor the confidentiality of the group
- To elaborate and expand on their own life stories

Individuals' Goals

The group goals, in most cases, complement goals that individual participants bring to the group. Individual goals might include the following:

- To learn more about oneself
- To find a greater sense of meaning in one's life
- To find some direction for the future
- To develop a sense of belonging
- To leave a legacy for the family
- To have fun learning, writing, and sharing

Leaders' Goals

Leaders and small-group facilitators who have already participated in the group process and have established personal goals will approach the guided autobiography group feeling less uncertain about their role in the group. Personal goals should be simple. The leader or facilitator should be able to achieve them without in any way limiting or inhibiting the natural development of the group. Some examples of leaders' goals follow:

- To arrive early to create a welcoming atmosphere (Avoid a sense of confusion or lack of preparedness by making sure that furniture is in place and materials are ready.)
- To greet individual participants by name as they arrive
- To encourage each participant to read his or her two pages (Warm, positive feedback will let shy participants know the leader and others are really interested in what they have to share. *Leaders should assure participants that they can skip parts they have written if they prefer not to share them aloud.*)

- To encourage each participant to interact with another group member at least once during each session (Leaders can encourage this interaction by noting similarities between stories and asking members to share similar or related experiences.)
- To promote bonding between group members by permitting them to interact freely within the guidelines of positive encouragement discussed in Chapter 5
- To encourage comfortable, spontaneous, positive feedback from group members, while being careful to ensure a fair distribution of time among participants
- To be sincere
- To avoid pressuring participants to discuss subjects with which they feel uncomfortable
- To be a trusted confidant and promote confidentiality in the group
- To listen attentively and acknowledge what is being said (This can be done in many ways. An open, comfortable posture, a nod of the head as someone speaks, passing a tissue if someone is on the verge of tears, or a paraphrase of something the person has shared all indicate attentive listening and acceptance. When appropriate, after a group member has read, the leader might comment on similarities with another person's story. This lets each member know that she or he has been heard and understood.)
- To refrain from offering interpretations of life stories (Interpretation is the responsibility of the individual who is writing the life story. The meaning of a life comes from within the individual; the leader merely provides the circumstances for its emergence.)

Recruiting Participants

Recruiting participants requires publicity. Leaders or organizations that wish to begin a guided autobiography program need to identify the potential audience and then promote the concept of guided autobiography to generate enrollment. If you are planning to conduct a workshop, in your advanced publicity you should be able to articulate the following points, in person and in writing:

- How you became interested in autobiography
- Why the Birren method of guided autobiography is a particularly help-ful means of discovering meaning in one's life
- How the workshop is structured
- The benefits of participating
- The dates, location, time, and enrollment information (including cost) for the workshop

Always include a phone number that people can call for more information.

Sponsoring organizations and group leaders might consider using some or all of the following publicity tools.

Networking

Network with individuals who have influence with the audience you wish to reach: ministers; administrators of adult education programs, school dis-tricts, hospital-based education programs, or counseling centers; out-placement and career counseling centers; your local library or bookstore; the local chapter of the American Association of Retired Persons (AARP); and so forth. You might prepare a cover letter with a concisely written proposal outlining the goals and structure of the workshop, and include, if you can, testimonials from people who have benefited from guided autobiography. Call to get the correct name and title of the person you need to communi-cate with, saying that you will be sending the course description and will call again after the person has had a chance to review it. Be sure to point out the reasons this program would benefit the members of the group you are trying to reach.

Creating Fliers

Create fliers to distribute to your audience. Make them visually appeal-ing, brief, and in large enough type to be read easily (see Appendix A for some examples). Break blocks of text into small segments that can be read and understood at a glance. Be sure to include the benefits of participating and the dates, time, place, cost, and a phone number for more information.

Point out that enrollment in the workshop is limited and participants will be accepted on a first-come, first-served basis.

Preparing an Article

Write an article for inclusion in your local newspapers or the newsletter of the sponsoring organization. In preparing the article, include the same kind of information as in the flier. Use a friendly, businesslike tone. Remember that a newspaper will run announcements but not blatant promotions. You can't say this is the greatest life-transforming experience on the face of the earth, but you can include an attributed complimentary quotation from someone who has taken the workshop. Be honest and sincere in your promotion. Say what you want to achieve in the workshop. Try to give readers an image or story that will stick in their minds.

Double-space your text and use active verbs, not passive ones ("Dr. Birren leads the workshop," not "The workshop is led by Dr. Birren"). Check your spelling. Vary the length of your sentences. Take out words and information that add nothing to your message. Appendix A includes a sample press release.

When the article is ready, find out the name (and its correct spelling) of the editor who will handle your announcement. Send the article directly to him or her by fax or by mail. Be sure to include that day's date, the issue date in which you would prefer the article to appear, and your name and phone number in case the editor wants more information. After a few days, you can call to confirm that the editor received the article and to ask whether he or she has any additional questions.

Giving Brief Talks

Prospective guided autobiography participants feel more interested and secure if they know who will be leading the workshop. If they know your face and have a sense of your personality and enthusiasm, they are more likely to enroll. One of the best ways to publicize a workshop is to speak for a few minutes at a meeting attended by prospective participants. For example, you might talk to the new members' committee at a church, to a meeting of a local chapter of the AARP, to a class on journal writing, or to the peer counseling class at a high school. Let them know why you are involved in guided autobiography, why they might find participation interesting or beneficial, and the details of when and where you will hold the workshop and how much it costs. Provide fliers with attached enrollment forms (see Appendix B).

Giving Abbreviated Workshops

Although the full, ten-week guided autobiography workshop offers greater opportunity for in-depth exploration of life history, shorter workshops can be an effective introduction. We found that a one-hour presentation at a church-sponsored women's retreat followed by an additional optional hour of writing and sharing generated enough interest for full enrollment in follow-up ten-week courses that included both men and women. Enthusiasm for guided autobiography spreads by word of mouth.

Adapting Materials to the Needs and Interests of the Group

The themes presented in this manual are appropriate for most groups. They are organized to move participants from general themes to more personal and sensitive themes as trust develops among group members and in the confidentiality of shared experiences. The final themes orient participants to the future. In some cases, especially in groups with specific group goals, leaders may develop and substitute themes that more closely support the goals and interests of the group. Examples of themes for specific groups are listed in Table 1. The leader can develop the appropriate sensitizing questions for these themes, or the participants can brainstorm to develop sensitizing questions as part of the group discussion. (See Appendix C for ideas on creating different themes.)

Table 1. Sample themes appropriate for specific groups

Type of group	*Special theme*
Vietnam War veterans	Impact of service on subsequent reintegration into society
Ethnic minorities	Impact of societal attitudes, political involvement, and ethnic identity in personal development
Prospective retirees	Productivity and interests outside work
Recovery groups	Addiction and its impact on self and others
Management team	Leadership style and its impact on individuals and the organization
Reading group	Interest in reading and the impact of books
Leaders	Sources of inspiration as a leader and as a participant
Church group	Spiritual life
Physicians	Medical practice and personal impact of recent changes in health care delivery

Scheduling the Time and Location of Group Sessions and Arranging for Facilities

The ten-week course includes ten sessions of two to three hours each, the time depending on the size of the small groups and thus the time required for small-group sharing.

Group Size

In the ten-week workshop, we find that twenty to twenty-five participants is a good working size. For the second half of each session, this large group breaks into smaller groups of five to six participants for sharing work and receiving feedback. Unless you have a room large enough to comfortably accommodate more small groups, or breakout rooms in addition to the large meeting room, you will have to limit enrollment. Small groups of fewer than five people may have difficulty discussing and sharing fully if one or two members are absent.

The format for one-day workshops is different. We have taught one-day workshops with more than a hundred participants. In such cases, the sharing is usually done in spontaneous pairs or groups of three or four people with no formal small-group facilitator.

Space

The space you use for the workshop should be large enough for both large- and small-group discussions. Acoustics are important because the simultaneous small-group discussions can generate a lot of noise. If you can find a room with carpet and draperies, the soft surfaces will dampen some of the white noise and create a homey, comfortable atmosphere. Avoid a formal classroom arrangement with all chairs facing the leader. A circular arrangement of round or rectangular tables creates a friendlier environment and encourages participants to interact with each other. For the large group, a tabletop or armchair writing surface is helpful. When the large group breaks into small groups for sharing, the small groups can sit at tables or in circles of chairs in different parts of the room, or if possible in different rooms. Possible sites for an autobiography workshop are a community center, library, corporate conference room, church facilities, or adult education classrooms.

Materials

A blackboard, white board, or flip chart and appropriate writing instruments are useful in guiding the direction of some of the large-group discussions. Participants will need blank paper and writing materials for some session exercises. Most people will bring their own, but you may want to have extras on hand. Participants almost always appreciate the availability of coffee, water, and other beverages. You might discuss in the first session whether people want to sign up to bring snacks for the group. This can be a nice touch, but remember, we live in a busy, health-conscious world, so don't force the issue if people don't want to bother.

CHAPTER 5

Small-Group Dynamics

*Each friend represents a world in us, a world possibly not born until they
arrive, and it is only by this meeting that a new world is born.*
—Anaïs Nin

*A friend is a person with whom I may be sincere.
Before him, I may think aloud.*
—Ralph Waldo Emerson

The Significance of Small-Group Work

Much of the transforming work of guided autobiography occurs within
the small group, when workshop participants share what they have written
at home.

Participants will already have discovered that writing needs more concentration and focus than simply remembering. In writing we have to make
decisions that require weighing the relative importance of events. We have
to choose what to write about and then stay with a thought long enough to
write it down. Often, participants are surprised about what comes to mind,
and they are startled by the significance these events have for them and by
the accompanying emotions. Reading the material aloud to a group of others who are sharing their experiences in similar fashion almost always takes
people to a higher level of insight and understanding than they can achieve
through the writing alone.

The confidentiality, trust, and empathy of the small group are so important to the success of guided autobiography that this chapter is devoted to questions of how to manage small-group dynamics. Some critical elements of success in small groups are

1. agreeing on common goals;
2. emphasizing confidentiality;
3. trying to maintain ideal group size;
4. carefully selecting facilitators;
5. judicious sharing by leaders and facilitators;
6. handling strong emotional reactions;
7. troubleshooting;
8. maintaining feedback between facilitators and the workshop leader.

Fostering Trust and Reducing Misunderstandings by Agreement on Common Goals

Trust within the small groups grows from participants' pursuit of common goals. For effective small-group interaction, all participants in a guided autobiography workshop must understand and support the structure of the workshop and be committed to the following goals:

- Refreshing and recalling the memories and events of their lives
- Organizing their life stories
- Sharing their life stories with others
- Attending all meetings, if at all possible
- Completing all writing assignments
- Listening actively when others are sharing in order to learn from their stories
- Offering supportive, encouraging, and empathetic feedback after group members have shared their work
- Avoiding interpretation or evaluation of what others read or say
- Avoiding comments or comparisons that imply judgment of the choices, feelings, beliefs, or opinions of other group members
- Respecting the confidentiality of all information shared in the group
- Enhancing everyone's enjoyment of the group by sharing time equally,

participating fully, and showing respect and concern for each group member

Advanced publicity should indicate that the guided autobiography workshop involves writing, reading two pages aloud in a small group at each session, and receiving supportive feedback from others who also are sharing their life stories. Sometimes people enroll in the workshop wanting to pursue self-discovery through personal writing alone. They are willing to write but are not yet ready to share their writing with others. Only individuals who share the personal commitments listed above should enroll. The strength of the group process depends on this.

At the first workshop session, the leader should discuss the basic goals, emphasizing the importance of adherence to these commitments for the success of the small groups.

The Confidentiality Issue: Revisit Frequently

The importance of confidentiality cannot be overemphasized. Trust in other members of the group is essential. Participants must feel as safe sharing their feelings and personal experiences with their small-group members as they would with a trusted friend. Sometimes participants will feel freer to share in a small autobiography group than in any other situation because of the understanding that they will not be judged and that what they say will not be repeated.

Size of the Small Group

The ideal small-group size is five or six people. This is large enough to include a diversity of experiences and variety of personalities, and the group will function well even if someone needs to be absent. In the small-group sessions, allow about fifteen minutes per person, about ten minutes to read and about five minutes for group feedback.

Selecting Small-Group Facilitators: Choose Carefully

Within each small group, someone should be designated to perform the following functions:

- *Managing time.* For everyone to have a chance to read and receive feedback, someone needs to watch the clock and gently give closure to one discussion and invite someone else to share.
- *Inviting interaction between group members.* The designated person can accomplish this by pointing out similarities between stories, pointing out similar strengths or creativity in the way participants dealt with situations, or asking a quiet member if the reader's story triggered other memories for him or her. This way of expanding the discussion should not take away from the reader, but should reinforce discoveries the reader has made through writing.
- *Troubleshooting* (see the section on this topic below).

Trained small-group facilitators who have already taken the guided autobiography course are familiar with the process and understand the depth of emotional reaction people often have to the themes. Their experience, when combined with good judgment and interpersonal skills, prepares them to handle situations that arise in group sharing. Paying for such assistance may be too costly for many sponsoring institutions. Several adaptations have worked quite nicely.

Paid Staff

An institution such as a Veterans' Hospital or a nursing home may allow paid staff to participate as small-group facilitators as part of their salaried positions. Ideally, these staff members will have trained as facilitators by taking an earlier guided autobiography workshop.

Trained Volunteers

Volunteer groups that serve hospitals, nursing homes, rehabilitation centers, cancer centers, schools, and other such institutions may be interested in autobiography and can be trained to facilitate the small groups. The best training is participation in an autobiography group with other volunteers.

Untrained Volunteers

From the roster of people enrolled in a guided autobiography workshop, the sponsoring institution may be able to identify a handful of individuals whose personalities and past experiences make them good candidates for facilitating small groups.

Rotating Volunteers

Sometimes the most practical solution for providing group facilitators is to ask each small group to select one member to act as facilitator for that session. This job can then pass to another participant at the next session.

Sharing Your Own History: Know What to Share and When

Leaders and facilitators can use anecdotes from their own life histories to prompt reflections and memories among workshop participants, always being careful not to upstage group members or step over the line into the role of dominant participant. In the small group, the facilitator's comments should be concise and supportive of group members' own discoveries and insights. For example, after a man shared a story about reconnecting with a brother after a long estrangement, the facilitator recounted the following.

It is a wonderful gift when siblings can redefine their relationship as adults. My sister and I were not close when we were growing up. I was the tall, quiet brunette, serious and studious with a handful of very close friends. She was blond and bubbly, a people-pleaser who was friendly with everyone she met. We cultivated our differences. But when we were young mothers, we lived near one another and began to share all the joys and pains, insecurities and triumphs of those years. We have so many interests in common. It was quite a revelation after all those years of competing! The intimacy has grown, and we are still best friends two decades later. A lot of things need to come together for a sibling relationship to shift. We were lucky.

The story does not compete with the one the group participant shared. It contains no judgment. It is just one person's story linking arms with another's, one person's insight and experience expanding another's.

In a different situation, this story might not have been appropriate to share. If the group member had described a reconciliation attempt with his sibling that failed, this story of a successful reconciliation would have been painful to hear. Leaders and facilitators must use sensitivity in choosing what to share of their personal histories, and when. But group members usually feel grateful to learn something personal about their guides. It strengthens the bonds of the group, gives the leader or facilitator credibility, and underscores the idea that even along the unique paths that individual lives take, we have many experiences and emotional responses in common.

The following are examples of personal anecdotes that are not intended to offer interpretations of someone else's life but to support a group member's story with another that shares common ground and reveals something the leader or facilitator learned from his or her own life. Injecting humor can also be useful. When sharing with their groups, leaders and facilitators should focus on the needs of the group, not their own needs, but they should also be honest about what they share.

Sometimes we can feel so angry at our parents because they seem to reject something in us that we value. People call me a free spirit. I am very enthusiastic and passionate about life. I love dance and art and am easily bored by routines. My father constantly told me to calm down. I hated that. It felt like he didn't like me. But now I realize he loved me, but I scared him. My grandmother (his mother) was like me, and she left my grandfather for another man when my father was only ten. My father didn't know that I wouldn't abandon him or that I would be a loyal and loving mother to my own children. He couldn't see that part of me because the side of me that soars scared him so much.

I was very chubby as a child. My brother and his friends called me "Fatty, Fatty, Two-by-Four." In early adolescence, I grew and slimmed down, but it took me a very long time to think of myself as something other than fat. In fact, I still struggle with that self-image.

I learned pretty early that one man's passion is another man's work. I wanted to be an archeologist because I thought archeologists traveled around the world to visit exotic places. Then I went on my first field trip in the Arizona desert. My professor put a pick in my hand and told me to dig. "Man, this is work!" I said, and I changed my major.

Handling Tears and Painful Memories

Some people feel uneasy about participating in a guided autobiography workshop for fear of the painful memories that may arise. Leaders and facilitators often feel uneasy about their ability to help people handle painful memories. Several factors guard against repercussions from the recall of painful events or feelings from the past.

Participants have control over their recall processes and what material they choose to write and share. The leader states clearly at the beginning of the workshop that participants do not have to share everything about their pasts. The leader might say, for example, "You may remember painful or even shameful events or feelings that you don't want to share. That is understandable. Just share what you are comfortable sharing. Sometimes, in talking about your past, you may unexpectedly feel sad or tearful. That happens to many of us." In this way, the leader creates a relaxed and tolerant atmosphere and gives individual participants a sense of control over what they write about and talk about in the group.

As the workshop moves forward and participants share more of the high and low points of their lives, trust grows within the group. Participants are likely to become more comfortable sharing memories of painful, regretted, or even unlawful acts, but individuals always retain complete control over what they choose to share. Group members usually respond naturally, showing supportive facial expressions, holding a hand, offering a tissue, or offering gentle verbal encouragement when someone suddenly or unexpectedly recalls an emotionally raw area.

Sometimes, a memory of something from long ago that did not seem to hold great emotional significance will produce unexpected tears, while another memory one has felt guarded about sharing may not be accompanied by any great emotional response when read to the group. In principle, we should not be surprised that some events of the past don't loom as painful as expected and others that seemed benign evoke strong feelings.

There are many different cultural responses to tears. They embarrass some people, whereas others find a place for them in everyday life. People who regard tears as a major happening will feel discomfited at their own tears or those of others and will want to rush to stop them. The leader should point out at the beginning of the workshop that sudden tears are not uncommon in guided autobiography. The experience is a bit like driving down a familiar highway and suddenly hitting an unexpected pothole that momentarily roughs up the trip, but then we move on. Tears are a reflection of the confidence and level of trust within a group. They should be neither encouraged nor discouraged but absorbed into the flow of the group.

Our minds are constantly making new associations. An elderly man wept in an autobiography group when he spoke of an incident in which his sister, now deceased, had wanted to do something with him when they were children, and he wouldn't let her. After stepping into this "pothole," he wiped his eyes and moved on to speak of other events. In a way, tears are a validation that one is getting into fresh material. Tears do not threaten an autobiography group. They usually make it stronger.

Sharing emotional and painful memories is part of guided autobiography. Powerful events, such as fires, floods, tornadoes, war, death, and separations, have touched the lives of many people. Such events leave important memories that should be recalled and integrated, with their significant facts and feelings, into one's life history.

The workshop leader should be at ease mentioning tears to a group. Acknowledge to participants that sometimes they may find themselves on the verge of crying when they think of something in the past. They should let it happen. It is normal and quite common in autobiography groups. Tell them to take their time and, when ready, to continue telling the story of their life.

Troubleshooting

This section offers some ideas for handling the most common difficulties in group dynamics.

Participants Who Dominate the Discussion

Some people will dominate the group discussion by talking too much or stating opinions in a way that inhibits other members of the group. Some possible solutions follow.

Divert the discussion to others. "Okay. We have heard from Esther. Let's see what others have to say."

Interrupt tactfully. "John, you are suggesting _____. Before we go on, let's see how others would like to respond to this."

Explain the importance of giving everyone time to read and give feedback. "Catherine, you and I are taking up quite a bit of time this session. Let's hear from someone else." Or, "You have made some interesting points or associations, and now we should give some other people an opportunity to speak." Or, if the person habitually dominates and is difficult to manage in more subtle ways, you can try saying to the individual or the group, "Let's pause a moment and notice our preferred style of participation. Some of us are listeners, and some of us are talkers. Let's each try to practice the opposite behavior and see what new things we can learn."

Participants Who Go off on Tangents

Here are some solutions to handling the situation in which people lead the discussion off track.

Bring the discussion back to the topic. "I think we were discussing _____ and have gotten a bit off track. Let's go back to our earlier discussion."

Recognize that a tangent can be worthy; if it is, give it some time before returning to the main topic. "This discussion is a bit off track, but it is related to our topic and seems to be an important issue for you. Let's take a minute to look at it more closely before we return to the main topic of our discussion."

Stop discussing the tangent. "This is very interesting, but we are way off the main topic of our discussion. Let's go back to _____. If any of you would like to explore this idea further, let's talk at the break."

Participants Who Do Not Write Their Two Pages

In any group, participants occasionally fail to write two pages for reading in the next session. Those who regularly don't write are usually anxious about their writing skills or have difficulty finding focus for their writing.

Permit people who have not been able to write to share their thoughts about the theme. Do this after all other participants have read their work and received feedback. Be sure not to let the person talk for more than ten minutes, about the same amount of time taken by those who read their prepared two pages. People who haven't focused their thoughts through writing have a tendency to ramble.

Remind participants of common goals. Writing two pages is a common goal stated at the beginning of the workshop. The writing focuses and sharpens thoughts about one's life before coming into the small group. Reading and sharing within the group often opens new insights. Failure to write diminishes the impact of the exercise for the participant who doesn't write and can waste the time and diffuse the energy of others in the group who do. Ask participants to reaffirm their goals.

Help participants focus. Guided autobiography stimulates so many memories for most people that they are amazed at how much they have to write. They want to write everything and have trouble narrowing their experiences to two pages, but this narrowing-down exercise is useful. When you look through a window or through a camera lens, you see only a partial view of the landscape, but the details within the frame have greater significance. If group members are having difficulty with focus, ask them to remember details or a vignette related to the theme and put a frame around it. If they describe what is in the frame, they will find the starting place for their two-page story. The significant details of their life history related to that theme will flow from there.

Shy or Reticent Group Members Who Slow the Energy of Discussion

There are several ways to encourage discussion by reticent group members.

Ask open-ended questions. Questions that begin with *what, where, why,* or *how* challenge group participants to expand their ideas and explain their positions more fully. Avoid questions such as "Do you think _____?" or "Is it true that _____?" or other questions that can be answered with very few words.

Find associations between the writing of a shy person and that of another person who has read. "Carl, you grew up in the Middle West during the Depression, too. How was your experience different from Christine's?"

Ask group members why they think the discussion is bogging down. Perhaps the theme is not moving all the participants. Perhaps people feel afraid or unsure of what is expected of them. Relaxed, nonthreatening discussion can bring these worries into the open. Assure participants that they can choose what they want to share. No one will pressure them to share confidences they feel uncomfortable discussing, but part of the guided autobiography experience is receiving support and positive feedback from other members of the small group. Help group members understand how they can provide this support for one another. Offer examples of positive feedback: "I think what you did took a lot of courage"; "I think I understand how you feel. I didn't get my height until I was eighteen. I always thought of myself as small and not athletic, too"; "What a riot! Look how your sense of humor helped you gain control in a difficult situation."

Group Members Who Make Negative or Judgmental Comments

The purpose of the group is not to make judgments about the past, and no group member should assume the role of social worker or therapist.

Reiterate the goals stated at the beginning of the workshop. The goal of small-group members is simply to help one another in this exercise of self-discovery. The prizes are richer recall of memories, new associations and insights inspired by these shared stories, and the gift of understanding—not a judgment of right or wrong.

Participants Who Are Experts on Every Topic

Occasionally, a group has a member who consistently considers himself or herself an expert on topics that arise during the reading and feedback.

Avoid argument and divert discussion. "I appreciate your point of view. Let's see what others think."

All Group Members Speaking at Once

There are a couple of ways to handle situations in which several people are speaking at once.

Use a flip chart to focus discussion. "Wait a minute. I hear so many interesting ideas. Let's get them down one by one so everyone can learn from them."

Emphasize good listening skills. "We may be missing a lot of good ideas. Let's practice good listening skills while we take turns speaking."

Participants Who Withdraw from the Group, Looking Displeased

Sometimes a group member shows by facial expression or body language that she or he disapproves of what is happening in the group.

Approach the person individually during a break. "I've noticed from your expression that you seem displeased with the discussion. Would you like to share your thoughts with me?" Or, "From your body language, I assume you are displeased with the discussion. How do you think it might have been improved?"

Participants Who Share Very Serious Material at an Early Session

Someone's sharing serious, dark material at an early group session can leave other group members at a loss for how to respond. Participants almost never throw in a blockbuster on the first day, however. If they do, they may be doing it to get attention. Or they may have been in a support group or in therapy and are thus more comfortable sharing deeply from the start. Usually the major repercussion is shock on the part of the other group members and uncertainty about how to respond. Here are some ideas on how the workshop leader or small-group facilitator can handle this situation.

Speak to the person privately or in the small group; express your understanding that the person is dealing with very serious, difficult issues. Emphasize that guided autobiography is no substitute for therapy. If it seems necessary, ask the participant to go a little more slowly in sharing this material. Other members of the group will most likely respond in a supportive way if they know how.

Model some appropriate feedback. Respond to the person's sharing with comments such as "Maybe your creativity was an escape for you. I can see why you like acting so much"; "What a source of comfort and kindness you were to your sister"; "It is hard to imagine anything more difficult for a child to face"; or "Thank you for sharing your story with us."

Provide a universal recap before moving on. After giving supportive feedback, point out to the group that we don't really know what life will present to us. We might find ourselves in an embarrassing situation at an inopportune moment, or we might experience a terrible loss, the uncertainty of emotional instability, the pain of abuse, or the thrill of an unexpected opportunity. Somehow we have managed to come through many ups and downs, and these stories—our stories of growth and survival—are provoking, no matter how simple or complicated they seem on the surface. Then ask, "Who would like to read next?"

Participants Who Act as Therapist

A group member who has a professional background in, experience in, or some knowledge of therapy may feel she or he can offer prescribed interpretation of another person's life.

Remind all group members that guided autobiography is not therapy and its purpose is not to interpret other people's lives. The goal of guided autobiography is simply to help people tell their life stories in everyday language. Any interpretation should come spontaneously to the individuals themselves as they integrate and write down the experiences that have been important in their lives.

A Small Group That Becomes Too Small

Ideally, because of the trust that evolves, small groups and their facilitators remain intact throughout the ten sessions of the workshop. But, owing to withdrawals or absences, an original small group may become too small to permit adequate variety and texture within the group. We have found groups to be very adaptable. When three people from one small group were absent, the remaining two simply joined another group. The guided autobiography experience seems to foster the supportive attitude and trust necessary to make such transfers workable.

Each Small Group Wanting the Attention of the Workshop Leader

The leader can participate in a different small group each week. This is less disruptive and more rewarding for both the participants and the workshop leader than the leader's floating to several groups in one session.

Participants Who Persistently Disturb the Work of the Group

In our experience, seriously disruptive or disturbed individuals do not usually enroll in autobiography workshops. However, group leaders and facilitators must be prepared to handle such a situation, should it arise. The disruptive group member might speak on an irrelevant topic, seemingly unaware of the flow of discussion in the group. He or she might carry on a long monologue that does not move the discussion forward, or show symptoms of mental or emotional disturbance.

On the occasion of the first disruption, the leader or facilitator might speak to the disrupting person in a mild manner, reminding him or her of the topic being discussed and the need to share time. If the disrupting individual repeats the behavior, the leader might speak to the person outside the group or by telephone, explaining that the purpose of the group does not seem to match the individual's needs. Express regret that the group is not what the person had expected but firmly suggest that the individual drop out of the workshop, since it is not serving a useful purpose. If possible, offer to refund any payment the individual has made for the workshop. If the person seems seriously disturbed, work in conjunction with your sponsoring organization or other appropriate authorities to refer the person to relevant professional or volunteer resources.

Remember that the primary purpose of a guided autobiography workshop is to encourage individuals who want to organize and share their life stories. The group should not become a victim of the dominating needs of an individual who requires outside help.

Getting Feedback from Small-Group Facilitators

It is very important for leaders to meet with small-group facilitators briefly each week—after the session, if possible, or sometime before the next session—to identify and address problems or opportunities that arise within the small groups. Also, at the beginning of each large-group session, it is wise to devote a few minutes to discussing participants' problems and concerns. Remember that the basis for any confidant relationship is good communication. You can't force trust or friendship, but you can create fertile ground where seeds will grow when the time and conditions are right.

PART II

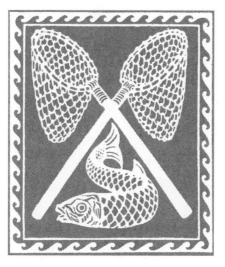

Session Plans

The Major Branching Points in Your Life

OBJECTIVES

Get acquainted

Introduce concepts of guided autobiography

Explain the organization and structure of the workshop

Begin to stimulate memory recall

Introduce theme 1: The major branching points in your life

MATERIALS

Flip chart, blackboard, or white board

Markers or chalk

Nametags

Enrollment List (Appendix B)

Plain white paper, pencils, and (if available) crayons

Handouts (Appendix B):

    Information Forms (or 3-inch × 5-inch cards)

    Workshop Outline

    Goals and Guidelines for Group Participants

    Rules for Group Leaders and Facilitators

    Theme 1: The Major Branching Points in Your Life

    Your Life Graph

    Leader's Life Graph, or Sample Life Graph in Appendix B

---

1. Preparation: Set a warm and welcoming tone

First impressions can be vital and lasting. To set the tone for the workshop, make the first session interesting, meaningful, and fun. Involve participants in interactive discussion and exercises that

1. sustain attention;
2. stimulate memories;
3. link the ideas you present to participants' own experiences;
4. encourage interaction among participants;
5. incorporate humor.

Arrive early enough to ensure that materials and seating arrangements are in order. If there is a flip chart or board in the room, write on it your name and, if relevant, the name of your sponsoring organization.

Fill in the Enrollment List with the names and phone numbers of preregistered participants. If there is a fee for the class, discuss in advance with your sponsoring organization how to handle payments for participants who have not preregistered.

Write these quotations on the board or flip chart or read them to the group (see step 5 below):

Life can only be understood backwards, but it must be lived forwards.
—Kierkegaard

*Since you are like no other being ever created since the
beginning of time, you are incomparable.*
—Brenda Ueland

Put a nametag at each seat for participants to fill out and wear during the session. Then be ready to greet people calmly and warmly as they arrive.

2. Introduction: Welcome participants to guided autobiography

a. Welcome everyone to the workshop
Introduce yourself and give some background on why you are interested in autobiography.

b. Take care of business
Ask participants to put on nametags. Circulate the Enrollment List. Ask participants who have not preregistered to add their names and phone numbers to the list. Ask everyone to initial the session date.

Hand out the Information Forms (or 3-inch × 5-inch cards) and ask participants to provide the following information:

- Name
- Street address
- City, state, and zip
- Work and home phone numbers
- E-mail address
- Age and gender
- Education level
- Major life work
- Name(s) of spouse or friends also enrolled in the workshop
- Goals for the workshop and an interesting fact about themselves (written on the reverse side of the form or card)

Explain that you will use this information to create a roster, to guide you in adapting the workshop to the group's interests, and to achieve diversity when assigning people to their small groups. Explain that heterogeneous groups (with diverse ages and backgrounds) take a little longer to develop rapport but are richer in the long run. Homogeneous groups tend to start off with enthusiasm but then run out of steam. If spouses or friends are attending the workshop together, put them in different small groups.

Collect the forms or cards and use them to create a roster and organize small groups for next week, and keep them for reference during the workshop.

c. Inform the participants about schedule and breaks
Tell participants how long the sessions will last, when the coffee break will be, and where restrooms are located. Express how pleased you are that they have come to embark on this journey of discovery with you.

d. Dispel anxiety
Recognize that people may be feeling nervous about sharing personal information, about their writing skills, and about whether they will feel comfortable and successful in the workshop. Share some stories from your own experience. One leader told the following story.

I remember on the list of required school supplies for second grade, the teacher asked each kid to bring two erasers. My mother thought that was excessive and bought only one. Have you ever watched second-graders? They are learning to write in cursive and they want to be absolutely correct. They write and erase and write and erase. When time came to turn in the first assignment, I had half an eraser, a paper with a hole in it, and no writing.

Tell participants that you don't want anything like that to happen to them. And because you don't want them to feel uncomfortable with writing or sharing, you are going to say a few things on these topics.

About the writing

In an address at Harvard Divinity School in 1838, Ralph Waldo Emerson said, "But speak the truth and all nature and all spirits help you with unexpected furtherance." Good writing is about truth. We all need and want to understand who we are, and writing and sharing our autobiographies help us with that. Professional writers who have taught autobiography courses are amazed at the quality of writing produced by people who have never considered themselves writers. Maybe this is because they are writing from the heart about things that are very important to them.

Most of our uneasiness about writing arises when the voices of our internal editors or critics are too loud or enter too soon, disrupting the flow of ideas before we get started. It may be hard to keep our editors from entering the room with us when we begin to write, but we can discipline them to be quiet and wait their turn, or we can learn to keep them in their place by viewing their antics with amusement.

As you talk to the group, encourage these budding autobiographers to write their life histories from the heart, without worrying about literary style. Tell them, "Just write as your mind flows, and keep your writing hand moving. Use simple, everyday English. Don't worry about spelling or style. Just write. Magic will happen."

About the sharing

The role of guided autobiography is to help people remember their stories and to organize them in a way that makes some sense to them and to others. This can be a very revealing and fulfilling process. Sharing these written stories with others takes autobiography to a level beyond writing. Even more magic happens as people come to understand their own lives better and experience how other people's stories trigger even more memories.

Explain to participants that what they choose to share is entirely up to them. They are the ultimate editors and no one may prod them to share more than they feel comfortable sharing.

NOW, HAVING LAID WORRIES ABOUT WRITING and sharing to rest, engage participants in an activity that will allow them to get to know one another.

3. Group exercise: Icebreaker activity

Purpose: To encourage participants to introduce themselves and begin interacting with one another.

First, write the following list on the board or flip chart:

- Name
- Birthplace
- Memory about a favorite childhood food

Ask participants to pair up with the individual on their right or left. They should take about five minutes to interview each other. Then, back in the large group, each participant introduces his or her partner by name, birthplace, and a memory that person shared about a favorite childhood food.

Next, get feedback on this process from participants.

- What do you think the value is of sharing personal information?
- How do you feel about people in the group now compared with at the beginning of the session?
- How did you feel when you heard others' histories and memories? Did their stories trigger memories in you?

4. Pose the question, "What is autobiography?"

Engage participants in interactive brainstorming on what autobiography is. Use the flip chart or board to list the group's ideas. Some possibilities:

- The story of your best friend told by your worst enemy
- A kind of timeline of events in a person's life

- A description of the matrix of events that compose a life (like creating a tapestry, interweaving many elements)
- A slice of a life history (a childhood, wartime experiences, etc.)
- A portrait of a friend, mentor, or family member who had an impact on your life
- A coming-of-age story
- A humor piece (a healthy, integrating way of coping with difficult material)
- An adventure story
- A love story
- Work history
- All of the above (sometimes we don't know what's there until our exploration of life history is well under way)

5. Pose the question, "Why write autobiography?"

Do some more brainstorming with the group about why one might want to write an autobiography.

- To leave a legacy for one's family
- To learn more about oneself
- To facilitate and understand transitions
- To enhance personal growth and development
- To achieve closure and a feeling of reconciliation about issues from the past
- To rediscover old interests and hobbies
- To find continuity amid the chaos and rapid changes of modern life
- To make new friends in a shared adventure
- To provide a history of a community

You can draw on your own experiences and reading as well as on the stories and background information in Chapters 1 and 2 to expand on these examples.

Now, draw attention to the quotations you have written on the board or flip chart, or read them to the group.

Life can only be understood backwards, but it must be lived forwards.
—Kierkegaard

We all seek an understanding of ourselves and answers to the questions, "Who am I?"; "Why am I here?"; "What makes me unique?"; and "How can I put my specialness to good use in my life?" We may find answers to these questions through life review. The answers we find tend to influence the way we view and live the future.

> *Since you are like no other being ever created since the*
> *beginning of time, you are incomparable.*
> —Brenda Ueland

This is a wonderful, affirming quotation for individuals to ponder as they begin the guided autobiography workshop. Brenda Ueland was a writing teacher who wrote a wonderful book called *If You Want to Write* (published in 1938). This book on writing and the creative process honors the courage it takes for individuals to come to understand themselves and put their words down on paper. Tell your workshop participants, "Your life stories tell what you have lived through. All of you are courageous, unique, and incomparable. You may not believe that now, but over the course of this workshop, you will come to believe it of yourselves and of your fellow participants."

6. Explain what guided autobiography is

Tell the group that guided autobiography is a structured means of organizing one's history. Hand out the Workshop Outline and tell participants something along the following lines.

The workshop will include ten sessions of two to three hours, with one ten-minute break. Each session will focus on a different life theme. The priming or sensitizing questions that introduce each theme assignment will help you think more deeply about how various aspects of your life history have helped shape you into the person you have become. Guided autobiography takes you on a more interesting journey, producing a more complete story than a simple chronology can. The themes and sensitizing questions act as a guide, just like a guide for a fisherman. They lead you to good fishing holes where the plump fish of memory are hiding.

The first fifteen minutes of each session are devoted to any necessary business or troubleshooting. This is followed by forty-five minutes of discussion related to autobiography and the session theme, which is your writing assignment for the next session. We then take a ten-minute break.

The second part of the session (one to two hours) is dedicated to small-group work in which each participant reads two pages of personal history related to the theme of the last session and receives feedback from other group members. Each person will have about ten minutes to read and five minutes to receive feedback. All feedback should be supportive and nonjudgmental. Often the feedback stimulates recall of more memories for the person who has just read, as well as for other participants.

During the ten weeks of the workshop, themes progress from relatively neutral territory to more personal subjects and finally to more present- and future-oriented topics. All participants have complete control over what they choose to share. No one should pressure any participant to reveal more than she or he feels comfortable sharing. Typically, in a good, supportive group, everyone becomes willing, over time, to take risks and share more deeply.

More than other approaches to autobiography, guided autobiography accommodates a view of life as a matrix with many different themes or threads that interweave as a life unfolds. Work, family, hobbies, interests, external events, emotions, and the people we meet do not act in isolation from one another. They interact in our lives in such interesting ways! Guided autobiography helps people explore the matrix of their lives.

7. Discuss the importance of confidentiality, trust, and having a confidant

a. Confidant relationships

Having a relationship with one or more confidants is important for people of all ages. Sharing fears, feelings, and insights helps us resolve issues in our past and present lives and see things more clearly. A good confidant relationship promotes insight and understanding and relieves stress, makes us feel loved and appreciated, and gives us vital feedback about who we are. People with confidant relationships are happier and physically healthier. We sometimes have a confidant at work or in some other specific area of life, but it is wonderful to have someone with whom we feel comfortable sharing all our thoughts and feelings, with confidence that what we share will not be retold elsewhere or held against us later.

Participants in an autobiography group enter into a confidant relationship with other workshop participants, especially the members of their small group. Trust is essential, and a confidant relationship is most successful if the sharing of confidences goes both ways. Fears often dissipate with trust and confidence in others, and trust grows if others are sharing similar material. Nevertheless, how much and what participants choose to share is entirely under their own control.

Share this quotation:

A friend is one to whom one can pour out all the contents of one's heart—chaff and grain together—knowing that the gentlest of hands will take and sift it, keeping what is worth keeping, and, with the breath of kindness, blow the rest away.
—George Eliot

b. Trust

Trust builds over time. You can illustrate this point using the analogy of airplane passengers. When you get on a plane, you might exchange pleasantries with the stranger next to you. If that person immediately pours out his or her whole life story with the most personal details, you are likely to want to escape, get your nose into a book, and share nothing of yourself. However, if one person shares a little information in a pleasant way, the other may share a little in return. Here is an example:

"You are going to need that heavy coat in Chicago. I hear it's snowing there."
"I hope the traffic isn't too bad. My grandson is picking me up, and he hasn't been driving long."
"Are you originally from Chicago?"
"Yes, I grew up on the South Side."
"Me, too. I attended the University of Chicago and left for California the day I graduated, but I still love the city. It still feels like home. I learned to drive in snow here, too."

In this way, if the conversation develops comfortably, the new acquaintances may feel a growing sense of trust and willingness to stay with the dialogue. Sometimes such a conversation can leave you with new ideas or thoughts that remain with you for a long time. Occasionally, such an exchange can be the beginning of an important relationship.

Or, you can illustrate the process of growing trust in another way. If one person puts down a nickel, the other person might respond with a nickel or a dime. Then the other person might respond with a quarter. If one party pulls out a $100 bill, the other may become anxious and pull away from the exchange.

Trust in a guided autobiography group grows in similar fashion, but more rapidly than in a regular encounter because the common goals and guidelines facilitate trust. Sharing personal stories in this safe setting quickly makes strangers feel as though they are among family or trusted friends.

8. Take a ten-minute break
Tell participants that after the break, the group will practice some sharing through an exercise aimed at stimulating memory.

9. Group exercise: Drawing a room from one's childhood
Purpose: To stimulate memories and illustrate the significance of details, especially details related to the senses.

This exercise was developed by the Reverend Carl Scovel of Kings Chapel in Boston and was featured in Dan Wakefield's book *The Story of Your Life: Writing a Spiritual Autobiography.*

Hand out pencils, paper, and (if available) crayons. Ask participants to draw a room associated with many memories from their early childhood. As they begin, start with the first instruction below, then gradually give the additional instructions, encouraging people to remember even more as they work.

- Draw the room, either as a painting or as a blueprint floor plan. Put in windows, furniture, rugs, curtains, or other furnishings that you remember.
- What decorations were on the walls?
- Add people you associate with this room. They can be stick figures.
- In the margins list the sounds, smells, and tastes you associate with this room. Do you associate music, special voices, or stories with this room?
- What about feelings and textures, heat, cold, special toys, or books? What games did you play here?

After allowing about ten minutes for this activity, ask participants to form groups of two or three to share the memories associated with their drawings. Take about ten minutes for sharing.

Back in the large group, discuss responses to this exercise.

- Were you surprised about what you did or did not remember?
- Did other people's sharing trigger more memories?
- Did you at any point feel the urge to begin writing?

10. Discuss the importance of small-group sharing

Describe how sharing within a small group enhances personal development through autobiography.

As we mentioned earlier, something happens in sharing memories with others that goes beyond what can happen with writing alone. Hearing others' stories helps us retrieve memories, things that had seemed forgotten. With feedback from others, we often can see our own stories in a different light or from a broader perspective. Our experience of history can actually change if our understanding of it changes. We may find resolution to troubling issues from the past. Through the sharing we see that everyone else has also had good times and bad. Everyone has dealt with adversity in some way and succeeded in coming through. The experience of sharing makes us more aware of our strengths and more optimistic about our future. The stories we share give us an expanded sense of what it means to be a human being. Setting group goals at the outset puts all participants on a common footing. Trust and comfort with sharing grow from this base.

11. Discuss the group's common goals

Discuss the goals that, no matter how diverse the group, provide common ground from which trust grows. Hand out "Goals and Guidelines for Group Participants" and ask someone or several people to read the goals aloud. Explain that when one or two people don't share these goals, it affects the whole group.

Ask if anyone has comments or questions about the goals or if anyone does not feel comfortable with them. Does everyone understand why these guidelines are important?

12. Discuss how small-group facilitators were selected

If you have trained volunteers or staff who will act as small-group facilitators, introduce them to the participants, explain how they were selected, and describe what their responsibilities are.

- To ensure that all participants have equal time to share and receive feedback
- To rotate the order of sharing so that the same people don't always start
- To facilitate the small-group interactions in a way that encourages balanced participation by all members; fosters supportive, non-judgmental feedback; and enhances recall of memories for all participants

If each small group is to select a facilitator each week from among its members, explain this to participants and hand out "Rules for Group Leaders and Facilitators." Ask all participants to read the rules carefully at home, bringing any questions with them to the next session.

13. Introduce theme 1: The major branching points in your life

Pass out the theme handout. Explain that branching points are those small or large events in life that turn us onto a new path and cause our life to take a new direction. A branching point might be a new school, a move, a new job, a marriage, meeting a new person, or even reading something that challenged you to think in a new way. Go over the sensitizing questions, emphasizing that these are to stimulate thinking. Participants should not try to answer all or any of the questions. Just considering the questions should help bring stories to mind. The questions are designed to prime memories.

Point out that often a branching point feels like an ending and then turns out to be the beginning of something new. This is what a *life transition* is—the loss of something known, a period of adjustment, and finally focusing on a new direction. Give examples from your own life to illustrate the kinds of stories that might be significant. Invite participants to join in the discussion.

Here are some examples of branching points.

When I was twelve, I came across the border from Mexico with some neighbors from my village. They brought me with them to Los Angeles, where I found little odd jobs for food. I would stay with one family for a while and then another, but no one I knew had any space or money, so I had to keep on the move. Finally, I got a job as a busboy and dishwasher in a restaurant and was able to pay a family a little to let me share a bed with their sons. I started to send a little money home to my mother in Mexico. At the restaurant, I learned that I could go to school for free at the local public junior high school, so I enrolled and worked at night. A counselor at the school found out about my story. I guess she could have sent me home, but she knew I was trying to do good for my family, so she took me under her wing and found me a permanent place to live. I was pretty determined to succeed in the United States, but without her help and encouragement, I don't think I could have finished high school or gotten the legal papers that enabled me to find better jobs.

When I was nineteen, I moved to Los Angeles to begin my college career. This was the most traumatic move of my life. I was unsure about going to college in the first place, and moving away from home made it that much worse. The night before classes were to begin, my dad almost had to shove me into the car. For a dime I would have stayed in Redlands and never, never pursued my college education. Today I am grateful my family was so adamant about my leaving.

When I was in graduate school, I had the opportunity to work on Robert F. Kennedy's presidential campaign. I remember he seemed so down to earth and really concerned about helping people. He wanted to do good work. Once I rode on the plane with him, and he came and sat with the students and reporters. Someone had a guitar, and Kennedy came and sang folk songs with us. When he died, I was devastated. I was supposed to be a delegate to the Democratic convention, but I had no heart for it. It seemed like the heroes were gone. I have not run for office myself, but have spent my career working behind the scenes in government and the private sector to help the poor and sick. Bobby Kennedy was a very significant role model for me. That branch was cut short, but others grew from the stub and were nourished by the same trunk.

The divorce of parents, the first day in a new school, a first date, learning to read, getting sick, losing a job—these are all branching points that may have more or less significance for one person than another, depending on many things, including age. Moving to a new school is certainly much different for a preschool child than for a teenager. Ask participants, "What were the significant branching points in your life? You don't have to mention all of them. Which were the most important to you?" Give participants a few minutes to list their branching points on a piece of paper.

14. Group exercise: Preparing a life graph

Purpose: To show participants that all of us have survived peaks and valleys.

Hand out "Your Life Graph" and be prepared to share your own life graph, which you have sketched before the session (Appendix B contains an example). Explain what the graph is and go over your own graph as an example. The graphing exercise asks participants to ascribe a positive or negative value to branching points. Point out that there is always forward motion with the passage of time. We pass through transitions. Some take us in a positive direction, some in a negative direction. Ask group members to mark their branching points at the appropriate age above the zero line for positive experiences (rated from 0 to 100) and below for negative experiences (rated from 0 to −100). Some experiences may have felt neutral.

Now ask participants to connect the points. The shape of the line reflects how we view our past branching points and begins to focus our attention on aspirations for the future. Tell participants to draw a vertical dotted line at their present age and to continue the lifeline into the future. How long do they expect to live? What kinds of transitions do they anticipate? Do they expect these transitions to be positive or negative? Of course, we do not really know, but it is interesting to speculate.

Ask participants to complete the graph at home and to use it as a tool in thinking about branching points. They can bring it with their writing to the next session to share in the small group.

15. Before adjourning, allow time for participants to ask questions and bring up any concerns

Let participants know they will probably have trouble keeping their writing to two pages, but that the two-page limit is necessary to give everyone time to share. If they write more, they can edit down to two pages or select two pages from what they have written. Editing to two pages results in stronger, more focused thinking and writing. Some participants write easily and will write a dozen pages a week. Others will struggle to write two. If a person has a disability that makes writing difficult, he or she can outline the main points and share from notes. Later, the person may want to dictate the autobiography in order to get his or her story fully recorded.

Suggest that participants find a quiet time and place where they can write for an hour or so without being interrupted. Ask them to review the priming questions and then begin to write with "I remember . . ." They should put down whatever comes to mind and write for at least thirty minutes. They should try very hard not to revise or edit as they are writing. That is a separate function to be done after the first draft is complete. If possible, they should set their writing aside for a day or two before coming back to refine it or edit it down to two pages.

16. Recap the tasks to complete before the next session
Instruct participants to accomplish the following tasks for the next session:

- Complete "Your Life Graph."
- Write two pages on branching points.
- Carefully review "Goals and Guidelines for Group Participants."
- Read "Rules for Group Leaders and Facilitators."

Your Family

OBJECTIVES

Improve memory recall through brainstorming techniques

Help participants feel more at ease with writing

Discuss participants' goals

Introduce theme 2: Your family

Introduce new ways of looking at family history

Initiate small-group work with ground rules

Share on theme 1: The major branching points in your life

MATERIALS

Enrollment List

Nametags

Flip chart or board and writing instrument

Small-group assignments (a card for each participant, with name and group number)

Handout (Appendix B):

Theme 2: Your Family

---

1. Greet participants by name, if you can

Ask all participants to wear nametags or create desk placards until everyone gets to know each other by name.

2. Get feedback on last week's writing assignment

Begin with a troubleshooting session. Ask how the writing went and give participants a chance to discuss any problems or obstacles they encountered. Ask questions such as the following:

- Did you have trouble remembering? Or did you remember so much you didn't know where to start?
- Did the sensitizing questions help?
- What questions would you add? Are there any you would omit?
- How did you decide which parts of your history to include?

3. Discuss problems of focus when one remembers too much
Focus is often a problem. People usually remember so much that they have trouble narrowing down the material they want to share to two pages. Explain to participants that choosing what to write is part of finding out what is important to them. Encourage them to tell the stories that *show* something about themselves and the people in their lives. "Show, don't tell" is the mantra of writing teachers. Anecdotes—just a few lines—can be very revealing. Say to participants, "You can't write about everything that happened over the years. Choose the incidents that illustrate a particular characteristic, the position or power a certain person had in your life, the incidents that meant the most to you." Encourage them to try *clustering*, a brainstorming technique borrowed from *Writing the Natural Way* by Gabriele Lusser Rico.

4. Group exercise: Clustering
Purpose: To reduce self-consciousness about writing and stimulate subconscious recall and the association of memories.

Ask participants to pick a color, let's say red. Write the word *red* in the middle of the flip chart or board and draw a circle around it. Then, as a large group, brainstorm for associations with the color red. You might end up with something like Figure 1. The cluster of associations that your group— or any group or individual—will create will differ completely from Figure 1 because the associations vary from person to person. In fact, an individual rarely comes up with the same cluster of associations twice. This doesn't matter. Clustering is a way of opening up thinking and letting feelings in.

Explain to participants that if they use this approach, they will at some point feel the urge to write. They will find focus, material, and direction. Ask them to try clustering on their own on a blank piece of paper: write the name of another color, then take five minutes to cluster and five minutes to write. Ask for volunteers to read what they wrote.

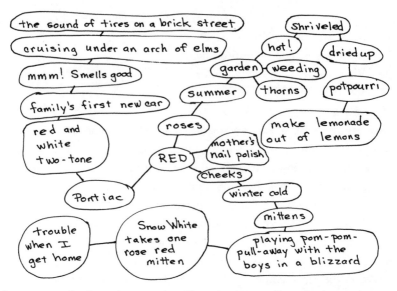

Figure 1. Sample clustering exercise. Clustering is a nonlinear brainstorming exercise that helps individuals remember life events through association of words, images, smells, and sounds. The process often puts writers in touch with more interesting subject matter than is possible through linear recall alone.

Suggest to group members that they do this at home with words related to the workshop themes, such as *family* or *work*.

5. Encourage participants to draw on all the senses

The five senses help us receive information. As children, before we had well-developed language skills, we depended on our senses of sight, sound, taste, smell, and touch to find out about the world. Sadly, we lose some of that "sensitivity" as adults. We favor sight over other senses. Through inattention, we lose some of the beauty of the world around us.

Encourage your workshop participants to try, as they write, to remember not only the sights but also the sounds, smells, tastes, and textures they associate with past events. Ask them to share some sensations that were important to them as children—the smell of wet mittens drying on a radiator, the twinkling of fireflies, the smell of freshly mowed grass on a summer night, the feel of fog on the face as one bundled up at the end of a day at the beach, the pain of cold toes crammed into ice skates that were nearly outgrown but had to last another season, the taste of fresh-baked molasses cookies.

Take any questions before moving on.

6. Ask how graphing the lifeline went

In a lifetime we face many branching points, or turning points. Some are presented to us by things beyond our control, such as natural disasters or health problems. Others are the result of conscious actions we take. Turning points are transitional times in life that usually involve some loss, some pivotal time to adjust, and then a sense of new direction. Ask participants if they can think of any transitions for which this is not true. Point out that even very happy, positive transitions involve loss and a period of adjustment. A new, loving marriage, a planned child, or a long-sought position of leadership—all very exciting and happy life changes—involve leaving something familiar behind. We can quite eagerly and happily adjust to something new, but we do have to adjust. The things we choose to leave behind and the ways we manage change are important elements in how we define our lives.

7. Discuss individual goals and expectations

Discuss the goals and expectations that came up on the forms or cards participants handed in at the first session. In most groups, quite a few participants are interested in completing a personal history to share with their families. Many come to the workshop for help in getting started on writing their histories and for the opportunity to share their journeys of self-discovery with others. Group members often produce very creative goals. One woman from a multinational family wanted to make a book of family recipes from the various countries represented in her family and include pages with anecdotes about family history.

Honor the goals of individual participants. Help them see how they can accomplish their goals through guided autobiography. For example, the woman who wanted to write a recipe book had planned to include only anecdotes related to food, but she ended up including stories that were not directly related to food but revealed important things about the character traits of family members and their interactions with each other. The ideas for her stories came directly from her writing on general life themes.

While recognizing that goals give us direction, encourage participants also to be open to whatever comes up as they explore various life themes in guided autobiography. The process of guided autobiography will help them recall material they might otherwise have overlooked. Spontaneity, humor, intuition, honesty, trust, and openness to personal insight help in the important phase of memory recall and self-discovery that supports strong writing. Overplanning the outcome can prematurely narrow our perspectives. Once we have access to our deepest memories and a way to organize them, we can present them in a variety of ways. Tell participants that in the final session, you will talk about ideas for completing and packaging an autobiography.

8. Introduce theme 2: Your family
Society presents a highly idealized image of family life that few, if any, of us experience. Most families are neither perfectly good nor perfectly bad. They cannot be described in black-and-white terms because they function with all the variety and nuances of Technicolor.

Encourage participants to write freely about their family histories from their own perspective. Ask if they have noticed that siblings raised in the same household often remember events from such different perspectives that they wonder whether they really did live in the same family! In a way, they didn't. Families grow and change, and each individual family member views life from his or her unique perspective. Workshop participants can write about their family of origin or their current family or both. People who now have no family can write about dear friends or pets who are like family.

Sometimes the figures we think of in a traditional nuclear family—mother, father, siblings—were not the most significant or influential for us. An unmarried aunt who led an interesting life as a career woman in the 1950s and who had time to shower attention on a favorite niece or nephew could have had a huge impact on the attitudes and development of that child. Sometimes a neighbor or close friend can function as a family member and be very influential. In a family with a child with special needs, that child can, without intending to, wield a lot of power.

9. Hand out the theme sheet and go over the sensitizing questions
Encourage workshop participants to use the priming questions to stimulate recall of memories and stories that characterize their families. Go through the priming questions as time permits, giving examples from your own life

and welcoming examples from group members to illustrate how much family structures vary. This is an opportunity for people to look at their families somewhat differently than in the past. Encourage an easy flow of conversation, but don't let a few people dominate. Keep the discussion balanced.

Invite participants to bring a picture of their family to the next session. They can pass the photograph around in the small group while they read their stories.

Here are some examples of anecdotes from family history.

On the surface, it looked like my father held the power in the family. My mother was very supportive of my father and all the family. My dad really acted like the head of the household. He ran a construction company and brought home the money. He was known for his intelligence and integrity and honesty and held a very high standard for all of us kids. He always asked us about our studies and our interests. When he came home late, no matter what we were doing, my mother insisted that we sit with him and talk with him while he ate dinner. Only when she died did we realize how much power my mother held. If Dad was the head of the family, she was the heart. She really helped Dad see the kind of encouragement we kids needed. I think she rounded off Dad's harsh edges. She cooked and sewed and was always there at home to listen to our worries and provide love. She was so soft and feminine, I thought she could never survive without Dad. Now I think she probably influenced every family decision. When she died, it was as if Dad had his heart ripped from his chest. I don't know how he survived those first years without her. She had so much more power than I ever gave her credit for.

My family expected a lot of me, since I was the oldest son. One of my family's strengths was their ability to keep me devoted to my education and not get distracted by sports or girls. At times that was a most difficult task! The members of my family were all busy with the requirements of their own lives, but they still showed me much love by word and deed. Throughout my life, whenever I saw or left either parent, it was always with a hug and kiss. Now, in retrospect, I feel especially blessed to have loving, kind, and understanding parents. I hope I have carried on the tradition. At least I have tried.

The story of my family is not all that wonderful because I never knew my mother or my grandparents on either side. My mother died of cancer when I was three. The powerful and key figure in my life was my father, a traveling salesman who was on the road six months of the year. I lived with eight or nine different relatives. I moved so much that it was difficult to form attachments. I didn't really have a family identity. I worshiped my father, who was tall and handsome. I always looked forward to his visits. When he was not selling garments on the road, his main pleasure was gambling. He was not an addict, but he had no other interests. He did not read books or plan for the future. When I was approaching thirteen, he asked if I wanted a bar mitzvah. We didn't belong to a temple, so I said, "I don't think so." He was relieved, but this led to a certain amount of shame and guilt over the years for me. Now I try to live my life completely the opposite of the way my father lived his. My wife and I are close to our family. Education is extremely important in our lives and none of us enjoy gambling.

My father knew my mother in grammar school. I know very little about their courtship. This is part of our family problem. We never discussed things. It also relates to my upbringing that I never felt it was proper to ask questions.

10. Recap the goals and guidelines for group participants

Remind group members that after the break, they will assemble in small groups to share their work. Take a few minutes to recap the guidelines or rules for group participants. Emphasize the following points:

- Read two pages of your life history.
- Listen attentively while others read or speak.
- Share only what you feel comfortable sharing and do not probe or prod others to share more than they want to.
- Avoid analysis, interpretation, or judgments of what others share. Instead offer supportive, encouraging, and empathetic feedback. Appropriate comments might be "I admire your sense of humor"; "You really showed persistence"; "You faced a lot of challenges and met them all with ingenuity." Not, "Your grandfather must have been nuts"; "You think that was bad. Let me tell you about . . . "; "Adult children of alcoholics often have this problem."
- Share time equally among group members in reading and discussion.
- Honor the confidentiality of all information shared in the group.
- Participate fully. What you get from the group is a reflection of what you give.
- Have fun!

11. Recap the role of small-group facilitators
Go over the responsibilities of the small-group facilitators.

a. Managing time
Each participant will have about ten minutes to read his or her work and five minutes to receive feedback. Facilitators should rotate the order of reading and sharing during the course of the workshop so that different people begin and end each session.

b. Inviting the interaction and participation of all group members
Facilitators should encourage all members to participate. Dominant members can be contained with comments such as "What you have said is very interesting. Let's hear what others are thinking." Quieter members can be invited to participate with questions such as "Mary, did Susan's story trigger any memories for you?"

c. Providing supportive feedback
All group members should provide supportive feedback, but the group facilitator must be attentive to the tone of the entire group, noticing the feelings and responses of the person who has shared and of other group members. If the discussion tends to wander or fragment, the facilitator can bring participants back together by paraphrasing, recapping, sharing an insight, or finding a universal theme. Here are some examples.

> *It seems like most of us were happier in transitions we initiated. To me, having a sense of control feels good!*

> *Mary, your compassion in caring for your grandmother seems similar to Jerry's compassion in caring for his developmentally disabled son. I admire you both and hope I have someone as loving to care for me if I need it one day.*

d. Troubleshooting
Facilitators must know how to handle problems that can arise in small groups.
   Tears and painful memories. One question that may trouble participants and small-group facilitators is how to handle tears and painful memories. Remember that group members share only what they want to share. As

trust grows, participants may feel comfortable sharing very painful memories. Even old memories that seemed to hold no great emotional significance can produce unexpected tears. Usually the other group members respond naturally with supportive facial expressions, holding a hand, or offering a tissue. Facilitators can tell participants, "Sometimes you may feel on the verge of tears when you think of something that happened in the past. Let it happen. It is normal and often happens in autobiography groups. Take your time, and when you are ready, move on with telling the story of your life."

If a group member gets emotional while reading, the facilitator should let him or her finish reading before offering supportive comments. Tears should be treated as a normal part of life and not as something unusual.

Other potential trouble spots. The most common sources of difficulty in a small group are unequal participation and someone who has a tendency to interpret or judge the work of others. Small-group facilitators should ask participants to help avoid these situations by taking personal responsibility for the welfare of the group. The facilitators should meet briefly with the workshop leader at the end of each session to provide feedback and identify any problems that have occurred during that session.

IF THE SAME SMALL-GROUP FACILITATORS will be leading all ten sessions, arrange to meet with them in advance of session 1. Share information in Chapter 5 on small-group dynamics. Do some role-playing for practice.

12. Assign people to their small groups
If the workshop has permanent small-group facilitators, introduce them and say which group number they will lead. If there are no permanent facilitators, designate a facilitator for each group or ask each group to select someone to watch the time and guide the discussion.

Hand out a card to each person in the workshop with his or her name and group number on it. This should go very quickly. Explain that people have been assigned to groups to achieve diversity, based on information provided on the forms or cards at the first session.

Emphasize again the importance of confidentiality.

13. Take a ten-minute break

14. Reassemble the small groups for sharing stories
Participants come back to their small groups to read their stories on theme 1: the major branching points in your life.

15. Recap the tasks to complete before the next session
Instruct participants to accomplish the following task for the next session:

- Write two pages on your family.

The Role of Money in Your Life

OBJECTIVES

Continue to foster self-confidence in writing and in the creative process

Discuss metaphor and the power of metaphor in autobiography

Provide basic writing tips

Introduce theme 3: The role of money in your life

Share on theme 2: Your family

MATERIALS

Enrollment List

Nametags, if still needed

Flip chart or board and writing instrument

Handouts (Appendix B):

    Writing Tips

    Theme 3: The Role of Money in Your Life

---

1. Greet participants by name and get feedback on last week's writing assignment

Take the first five or ten minutes to answer questions and address problems or insights people may have had in writing about their families. Pursue the discussion with the following questions:

- Did you try clustering?
- How did it work for you?
- Were you surprised at which stories came to the forefront of your memory?

2. Provide some writing tips

Sometimes at this stage, participants ask for tips to help make their writing stronger. While guided autobiography is not concerned with style as much as content and insight, the following tips can help make the writing easier and thus make the process of writing a life story more enjoyable. Some participants ask for tips; most appreciate them.

a. Writing with the right and left sides of the brain

The right side (or hemisphere) of the brain is more playful, seeks patterns and design, and is the seat of creativity. The left side is more analytical and likes facts, details, and rules. In writing, you may first write from your intuitive, spontaneous soul and later edit with your analytical mind. A good tip from Natalie Goldberg, author of *Writing Down the Bones,* is to keep your hand moving. Don't stop to let the "editor" in until you have finished your two or more pages.

b. Trusting one's creativity

Everyone is creative and needs to exercise that creativity every day. People who do this tend to become happier, less rigid, and psychologically healthier. Creativity never leaves us entirely, but unless we use it, it becomes more difficult to access. Cherish your creativity. Another word for creativity is *playfulness*. Children usually do not use toys in exactly the way they were designed to be used. They invent ways to play. For participants in an autobiography workshop, creativity may manifest itself in innovative ways to solve business problems, fix a car, market a product, comfort a child, create a sculpture, compose a photograph, design a flower bed, set a table, or write on a theme.

Encourage participants in your workshop to look for ways in which they have been creative in writing their stories without becoming too self-conscious or having their stories sound contrived.

Being creative is more or less a process of learning how to get out of one's own way. People can learn to be more playful and think about things in new ways. We have to learn to silence our inner critical voices that make us fearful. We all have these inner voices that tell us to behave according to the rules and not to risk ridicule by being different. Ask participants to think of life review as an exercise in self-discovery. Encourage them to treat themselves as gently and lovingly as they would a child. Tell them, "Go for it! Have fun! There are no wrong answers."

c. Using metaphor to communicate information and foster creativity

A metaphor is a figure of speech that uses a word or phrase denoting one kind of object in place of another to suggest a likeness. One woman in a guided autobiography workshop said she used to be a kitten, but now she had become a tigress. She upgraded her metaphor to reflect a new self-image.

Metaphors require *divergent thinking*, a process that generates alternative views or solutions to problems or questions. Our educational system tends to emphasize the development of convergent thinking—one and only one correct answer. Humor tends to rely on divergent thinking.

> *The lion went through the jungle roaring at all the animals, "Who is king of the jungle?"*
> *"You are," said the monkey. "You are," said the gazelle. "You are," said the hippopotamus.*
> *Finally he asked the elephant. The elephant picked up the lion in his trunk and threw him into the water. The lion came up sputtering and said, "Just because you didn't know the answer doesn't mean you have to get so mad!"*

This joke uses divergent thinking to make fun of convergent thinking. Convergent thinking has been overemphasized throughout the Industrial Age to prepare a specialized workforce for an economy based on mass production. Henry Ford didn't want someone on the assembly line daydreaming about what would happen if a wheel were attached in a different way. He wanted the wheel attached in exactly the same way every time.

Divergent thinking, however, makes us more adaptable, both in the modern workforce and in our nonwork life. Willingness to look at things from a new perspective opens our minds to creativity and change.

Metaphors are only a tool and can change as we change. Feedback from members of small guided autobiography groups will help participants think more divergently about themselves and their life experiences. Openness to alternative points of view helps us all in our writing and in our journeys through life.

d. Group exercise: Practicing with metaphors

Purpose: To encourage participants to broaden the ways in which they view themselves.

Ask participants to write down the name of an animal, flower, or object that they consider a good metaphor for who they are. Share these ideas in the large group, encouraging participants to explain why they selected their metaphor. Here are examples from past workshops.

> *I am an eagle because, like the eagle, I like to fly alone, high in the sky where I can get a better view of what is going on in the world.*

> *I am like a Sequoia. Day by day, my life doesn't look very exciting, but little by little, I grow, and many smaller people in the forest depend on my seeds and shade.*

> *I am a bridge. It seems as if I'm always connecting different cultures and bringing people together who otherwise might never meet one another.*

e. Using humor: It's healthy and creative

Learn to lighten up. Humor, as illustrated by the joke recounted above, is a form of divergent thinking. Humor helps us tolerate pain, release tension, and achieve biological, social, and psychological balance. That bodes well for our general health. Session 6 includes more about the use of humor in guided autobiography.

f. Staying relaxed about the writing

Tell participants not to get too uptight about writing style. Encourage them to relax. Tell them, "Guided autobiography is only a tool to help you gain access to the stories you already have inside you. You don't have to make anything up. Clustering helps you start from the left side of the brain where many of us feel more comfortable. From the collection of details, the right side of the brain sees a pattern, a direction, and a place to begin to write. Clustering creates a comfortable partnership between both sides of the brain."

g. Following some basic writing tips

Hand out "Writing Tips" and go over the tips in the large group.

3. Group exercise: Writing with pictures

Purpose: To give participants experience painting a picture with words in a short time frame.

Ask all participants to write for ten minutes about a person who was important to them in their adolescence. Encourage them to use metaphor and paint a picture with words. Ask them to help us *see* the person they are describing and know something about his or her character. Tell them to keep their writing hand moving for ten minutes. Then ask for a few volunteers to read what they have written. Provide positive feedback when metaphor, use of the senses, and concrete detail bring the writer and the listeners closer to the subject.

4. Introduce theme 3: The role of money in your life

The role of money is a loaded topic, somewhat taboo in many circles but very important in both obvious and subtle ways. It has an impact on many aspects of our lives: family, education, careers, health, relationships, and self-esteem.

Tell workshop participants that, in the course of the workshop, they will see some overlap between topics. They may find themselves revisiting issues they have brought up in previous themes. This is fine; it is part of the process of integration.

5. Hand out the theme sheet and go over the sensitizing questions

Discuss the sensitizing questions for this theme, giving examples from your life and engaging the large group in discussion as you have in the previous sessions. Here are some examples from the work of past participants.

No one among my relatives seems to have worked for financial reward alone. The family ethic was service. Find a way to serve people, and you will find yourself making a comfortable living. I recently have been thinking about my wife's family and how differently they think about work and money. A number of her relatives have been highly successful in business. Their ethic seems to be to concentrate on accumulating wealth, then they donate time and a portion of their assets to charitable causes—for education, the needy, and civil rights.

Growing up in the Depression had an effect on my attitude toward money. Unlike me, my children think nothing of talking at length on the telephone long distance. They readily valet-park while I look for a spot to self-park. I am still shocked at paying seventy-five cents for Lifesavers that used to cost a dime. My wife is like me. For years we got practical things for each other for our anniversary. Thanks to my career in banking, I am a good money manager. Money is not important to me except that I would like to have enough to continue charitable endeavors. Contributing to the community gives me a sense of value. When it comes to money, I subscribe to that old saying, "There are no suitcases on the hearse."

There was a strange paradox about money in my family. On the one hand, my parents taught us that character and kindness were better measures of a person than wealth. But at the same time, we had a feeling that we never had enough money. My parents were always worried about financial security, so money was very important. It was a subject that hid behind the curtains and breathed heavily.

6. Take a ten-minute break

7. Reassemble the small groups for sharing stories

Participants come back to their small groups to read their stories on theme 2: your family. If there are no permanent small-group facilitators, designate facilitators or ask each group to appoint someone to watch the time and guide discussion. Ask small-group facilitators to meet with you briefly after the session to touch base and troubleshoot. Do this at the beginning of small-group sharing for all subsequent workshop sessions.

8. Recap the tasks to complete before the next session

Instruct participants to accomplish the following task for the next session:

- Write two pages on the role of money in your life.

Your Major Life Work or Career

OBJECTIVES

Discuss the role of autobiography in personal development

Discuss self-image and how it evolves through feedback and experience

Identify the role of autobiography in integrating aspects of self-image

Identify some dimensions of self that contribute to self-identity

Introduce theme 4: Your major life work or career

Share on theme 3: The role of money in your life

MATERIALS

Enrollment List

Flip chart or board and writing instrument

Handout (Appendix B):

Theme 4: Your Major Life Work or Career

---

1. Get feedback on last week's writing assignment

Take a few minutes to get feedback from the large group about last week's writing assignment. Then introduce the topic of self-image and use the questions listed below to guide the discussion.

Self-image is very much a part of personal history. The events and people in our lives help shape our self-images, and our self-images, in turn, have an impact on how we react to people and life events. Self-image is dynamic and usually changes as we mature.

- How central to your self-image has your work life or financial status been?

- How has the importance of work life or money changed for you over time?
- Where did your attitudes about the role of work or money in your life come from? Personal values, family, the broader culture?
- What other kinds of things influence the image (or images) we hold of ourselves?

Validation or negation from other people in terms of our job, income, social status, physical attractiveness, creativity, intelligence, competence, or other measures of personal worth can be very powerful.

2. Discuss how autobiography can enhance self-awareness and personal development

Child development emerged as a field of study in the first quarter of the twentieth century. Children go through identifiable stages of development on their way to adulthood. What happens to them at each stage of development can either help them mature or impede their development in various ways. Our age and the stage of development we are struggling with when certain events occur can be very important to our future development.

Since 1900, the average life expectancy in the United States has increased from forty-seven to about eighty years, which means that the average adult now has *three more decades* of life. Interest in child development has expanded to include the whole span of human development. We continue to go through developmental stages from birth to death, and, as long as we retain our cognitive abilities, we do not lose our capacity to learn, to change, and to integrate our life experiences.

Personal development requires some awareness of the self. The trouble is, self-image can be pretty complicated and contradictory. We have many selves to integrate as we grow up and grow old. Through an often subconscious process, we develop self-identity through analyses and revisions of three versions of self-image: the ideal self, the social self, and the actual self.

Draw the model in Figure 2 on your board or flip chart as you begin this discussion.

The *ideal self* is the image of the person you would *like* to be. (A teenage girl might see herself as an anchorwoman on national television news, for example.)

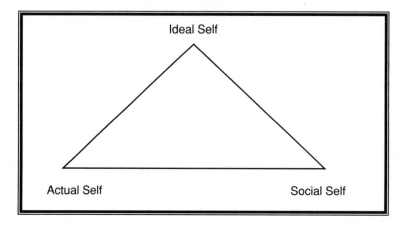

Figure 2. Three concepts of self. Self-concept is dynamic. We may feel confused by incongruity between the way we would like to be (ideal self), the way we believe others see us (social self), and the way we think we really are (actual self). As we mature and receive feedback from life, the points of the triangle tend to come closer together. The three versions of self become more similar, so we feel more grounded. Guided autobiography can be a valuable tool for integrating these three concepts of self.

The *social self* is your image of how others view you. (The teenage girl believes others see her as a dim-witted social butterfly.)

The *actual self* is the way you think you really are. (The teenage girl knows she is bright, but she is afraid to show her intelligence because smart kids are not highly valued in the social hierarchy of her school. She is struggling to reconcile feelings of insecurity with her ambitions and current image in her circle of friends.)

A Roman Catholic priest of our acquaintance has a print in his office that captures the tension of this triangle. In the lower right corner, a monk is standing in front of an easel on which his unfinished painting of a cardinal of the Church rests. The monk is holding his palette and brushes in one hand while he scratches his head with the other. On the easel, the canvas portrays the prelate dressed in his red robes looking very dignified and powerful. To the left, beyond the easel, is the actual cardinal posing for his portrait in a golden chair; he is plump and slumped in sleep, looking like a very ordinary human being. The dignified portrayal of the cardinal on the canvas is the ideal self, the sleeping cardinal is the actual self, and the monk's puzzlement represents the social self. The incongruity between the three versions of the cardinal creates a tension that is amusing in the picture but uncomfortable in life.

Disparity between our ideal, actual, and social selves tends to diminish with age. The actual self develops skills and competencies, the ideal self becomes more realistic, and the social image becomes truer. The highest degree of self-actualization occurs when these three selves converge. A big divergence between these three models of the self creates anxiety and discomfort. A lot of the volatility of adolescence results from the great disparity that still exists between the ideal self, the actual self, and the social self.

Feedback from friends and life experience, including guided autobiography, tends to bring the three versions or images of the self closer to convergence.

3. Group exercise: Changing self-image
Purpose: To illustrate that self-image is not a permanent condition but changes over time with feedback from life and friends.

Ask participants to draw two large triangles on a piece of paper. Then ask them to describe in a sentence or two their ideal self, actual self, and social self as an adolescent on one triangle and as they now are on the other. What kinds of experiences have caused the change? Ask participants to share in pairs or ask for volunteers who would like to share with the large group.

4. Brainstorm on the dimensions of self that contribute to self-identity
Ask the large group for ideas on aspects of self-identity and list them on the board or flip chart. Some examples:

- Physical appearance
- Intelligence
- Strength
- Vision
- Sexual attractiveness
- Sense of fun, pleasure
- Vulnerability
- Responsibility
- Athletic ability
- Accomplishments

- Creativity
- Position in the family (first, youngest, or middle child)

5. Ask participants what characteristics best describe themselves

Tell participants to write down five characteristics that best describe themselves, then ask them to circle the one they think is most true. Ask people to share their "primary" characteristic if they feel comfortable doing so. List them on the board or flip chart. Point out that most characteristics are likely to be positive. Explain that in the process of writing and receiving feedback, people may discover other very strong characteristics that will alter or expand their self-image. Ask them to save the list and do the exercise again near the end of the workshop, so they can compare the lists.

6. Introduce theme 4: Your major life work or career

People usually think of a career as something they do outside the home for pay, but that isn't necessarily their major life work. Our major life work is whatever occupies most of our energy, time, and attention or the activity we feel most passionate about.

A real estate agent was lukewarm about her career for many years until she found satisfaction in working as a volunteer in her church community. There she found a niche that gave her a sense of purpose and belonging. Her volunteer work became her major life work, even though she continued to sell real estate. In fact, many of her listings and prospective buyers came through her contacts with the church. She began to view her job not just as selling property for commission but as a mission to match families with houses that would suit their lifestyles. She found more satisfaction in her job when her goal was not only to make money but also to use her skills and knowledge to help buyers and sellers achieve their life goals. A history of this woman's life work would not have been complete without information on her volunteer work.

One's major life work could be a consuming hobby, such as writing or art, crafting, or volunteer work. It could be raising a family, supporting a spouse, coaching sports teams, or local politics, or it could be one's career or work-for-pay life.

7. Hand out the theme sheet and go over the sensitizing questions

In going through the sensitizing questions for this theme, give anecdotes from your own experience and solicit examples from group members to illustrate lines of thought that might be appropriate. Here are examples from previous workshops.

> *My life's work began at age three when I drew tombstones from advertisements produced by my father's employers. He was a salesman. My parents wrote names on my tombstones and used them as place cards for dinner guests. I also drew panels with simple characters acting out stories from my mind. I kept doing that for sixty-two years until I retired from writing and designing movies. Illustrating my own ideas was my first and lifelong aim. It was work well worth doing.*

> *I guess I have been a mother longer and with more dedication and investment than anything else in my life. Strange, but if anyone else had told me that was my career, my feminist hackles would have gone up, and I would have vehemently denied it. But since I came upon that idea myself, it must be so.*

> *I modeled for department stores and Simplicity Patterns. My father was in the garment business, but he wouldn't help me. My father had a saying that has been important to me throughout my life: "First people look at you. Then they listen." It always rang true for me. When you meet someone for the first time, in business or in life, before you get to know them, they have already formed some kind of opinion about you.*

> *My parents advised me that a married woman only needed a teaching credential as a life insurance policy. It was something to be activated in case of her husband's death. I taught school for one year. Later, I started a flower business. In 1976, I became a public affairs intern at City Hall. I later was asked to head a program to help victims and witnesses of crimes. I developed staff protocols and procedures and learned everything I could about witness assistance programs. It didn't occur to me that I was developing job skills along the way. I only thought about helping people.*

8. Take a ten-minute break

9. Reassemble the small groups for sharing stories
In their small groups, participants share on theme 3: the role of money in your life.

10. Recap the tasks to complete before the next session
Instruct participants to accomplish the following task for the next session:

- Write two pages on your major life work or career.

Your Health and Body

OBJECTIVES
Discuss the importance of both continuity and change in life history
Present perspectives on direction in human development
Establish the role of autobiography as a tool for integrating life
experiences
Introduce theme 5: Your health and body
Share on theme 4: Your major life work or career

MATERIALS
Enrollment List
Flip chart or board and writing instrument
Handout (Appendix B):
    Theme 5: Your Health and Body

---

1. Get feedback on last week's writing assignment

After taking any questions or comments on last week's writing, use the following questions to guide the discussion with the large group:

- Do you find that remembering stories from your earlier life raises questions about the context in which the events took place? Why did people
  do certain things? Why did events affect you in a certain way?
- Have you found that people whom you had not believed were influential in your life have, nevertheless, affected how events in your life
  unfolded?

Part of gaining wisdom is expanding our understanding of the broader context of life's events. While we are talking about family, money, work, and other subjects that sound mundane on the surface, we actually are writing a story of the experiences and moments of grace and insight that reveal to us who we are.

Make the point to group members that, while we are changed by the experiences we have throughout our lives, we also have a sense of continuity that is valuable. Tell the group, "Isn't it miraculous that with all the people who cross our life paths and with all the bumps and turns that shape our lives, there survives inside each of us a kernel of something authentic, unique, and consistent? Some things that were true of us as children remain true throughout adulthood."

Explain to group members that, in their writing, they will see progression and development but will also rediscover the authentic essence of themselves that winds through all their experiences.

2. Discuss ways of looking at directionality in life

There are many ways of looking at the direction of development in our lives. Some examples are the biological, social, and integrated perspectives. Sketch the graph in Figure 3 on the flip chart or board as you discuss these perspectives.

a. Biological perspective

The biological model illustrates physical development, the rise, peak, and decline of the average human body over a lifetime. We start as embryos, grow and develop through childhood, reach a physical peak sometime in our early thirties, then decline as we grow older. In part, the expression "over the hill" comes from this way of looking at human development.

b. Social perspective

The social model illustrates a view of human development that predominated through the early part of the twentieth century. Its influence is still evident in many of our attitudes and institutions. After birth, the line of development rises through childhood. Then, at about age twenty-one, the line flattens out and sustains a constant horizontal throughout adulthood. We are born as clean slates, spend childhood becoming educated and

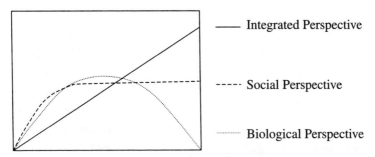

Figure 3. Three perspectives on human development. An individual might view the direction of his or her development as a human being in many ways. These are three examples: the biological, social, and integrated perspectives.

socialized (learning skills and manners), then spend our adult years in a fairly constant, stable state using our skills to support societal values.

c. Integrated perspective

The line of development in the integrated model rises steadily from birth to death. Throughout life, from birth to death, we gain knowledge, wisdom, and understanding through a process of integrating life experiences. We keep getting better. Our work is never done, our learning never finished, but the best news of all is that we are never "over the hill."

OF COURSE, REAL LIFE IS NEVER THAT SIMPLE. For many persons, life events and personal development may feel random and chaotic. Things may seem to be going along evenly for a while, then life takes a sudden upward or downward turn. Ask participants which perspective most closely resembles their view of life.

3. Discuss how some aspects of "self" develop more fully than others

Not all aspects of the self develop equally. This differential development may be due to life circumstances, the models we have had, our cultural backgrounds, or personal preferences. Share this Indian proverb:

Everyone is a house with four rooms—a physical room, a mental room, an emotional room, and a spiritual room.

As in most houses, we tend to use some rooms more than others. Some-times we close and lock the door to one of the rooms, blocking memories. Repression is one way of coping with difficult memories. All of us probably use repression, denial, fantasy, or humor to reduce difficult situations to some-thing that feels more manageable. The problem is that if something triggers a memory, even years later, we may snap back to the emotional state we experienced when the remembered situation took place. We feel fifteen years old and personally wronged all over again. To overcome this "developmental arrest," we can use memory to reinstate the old emotional state. Metaphori-cally, we can open the door to that room and let in the light. By reinstating the old emotional condition and letting in new information, we often can change our interpretation of events and, finally, lay them to rest so we don't have to keep those memories hidden behind closed doors.

Guided autobiography invites us to open all the doors and windows to let light and air into our whole house. We invite old stories to come forth from all the rooms. Then, when the stories go back to their resting places in our memories, maybe we will feel more comfortable leaving the doors and windows open so we can incorporate what lies in those rooms into our daily lives and live as more complete people.

4. Introduce theme 5: Your health and body
Health and body image is a sensitive topic that involves both the facts (height, weight, color of hair, color of eyes, etc.) and our subjective perceptions: how we view ourselves in comparison to others.

5. Hand out the theme sheet and go over the sensitizing questions
In going over the sensitizing questions, give examples from your own life, when appropriate, and draw members of the large group into the discus-sion. Here are some examples from previous workshops.

> *As a young boy, I was of average height, but in my mother's eyes, I was very skinny. She tried every way to put weight on me, but to no avail. Now that I have achieved senior status, my body image has changed. I don't know how I put on those forty extra pounds. I have gone from a well-proportioned male adult to a pot-bellied senior citizen. My belt has fallen below its proper horizontal position on my waist, and my butt has somewhat caved in.*

I think my sense of humor and above average self-esteem have helped me conquer difficult times. When my stress level rises, I somehow find more energy and resources to pursue my activities with renewed vigor.

My most serious health problem, and the one I live with every day, is being diabetic. When I was seven months pregnant with my second child, the doctor discovered that I had gestational diabetes. I spent five days in the hospital and learned about diabetes and how to give myself the insulin shots that I would need for the rest of my pregnancy. I had a third child, with diabetes present throughout the pregnancy. Since my early forties, diabetes has been a part of my daily life. I had to really re-evaluate my self-image. I had always been full of energy and never took pills, not even aspirin. Now I have to take multiple medications. For a while I lived in denial, but as the years passed, I took more control over my condition. In many ways, it has changed my outlook on life. I have seen the ravages of this disease and no longer expect to be among the old old. Instead I try to live each day and find pleasure in the things around me. I worry most that my children will inherit the disease. Each year that goes by that they don't get it is a good year for me.

When I was young, girls didn't participate much in sports. It was considered almost unfeminine. That was just fine with me. I considered myself very unathletic. Then, in the Kennedy administration, physical education became a requirement. I remember in high school on the first day of each school year I was first pick for the basketball team because I was very tall, but the second day I was always picked last. I had been found out. I always close my eyes when a ball comes at me from overhead. Now, as a mature woman, I know that there is more to athletic skill than catching a ball. I love to ski and hike. I am a pretty good dancer, and, in fact, as I look back now, I was a very active child. Maybe I am somewhat athletic after all, and my image of femininity has expanded enough to accept that without conflict.

I have been an athlete all my life and many times walked pain off to get back on the playing field. I love sports and was always proud of being a jock. Team sports taught me a lot about life, how to work with other people, give and take. I became a staunch believer in mind over matter. I was tough. Now I have had several surgeries on my knees and none have worked. My knees are shot. Walking, stairs, the exercise bike, everything hurts. I am struggling with too much weight and can't work it off. I hate not being able to do what I want to do. I still put mind over matter a lot, but it doesn't get me as far as it used to.

Ask participants, "Can you see how the writers are integrating new in-formation about themselves as they mature?" The image we have of our health and body has a big impact on all aspects of our self-image—the ideal self, the social self, and the actual self. Ask the group the following ques-tions:

- How have your health and body developed?
- How have they changed over time?
- Are your ideal, social, and actual health and body images more similar now than they were when you were a teenager?
- Where does feedback on your health and body image come from?
- Why are we so sensitive about this aspect of our self-image?
- How closely are your physical health and body image linked to your sexual identity?

6. Take a ten-minute break

7. Reassemble the small groups for sharing stories
In the small groups, participants share on theme 4: your major life work or career.

8. Recap the tasks to complete before the next session
Instruct participants to accomplish the following task for the next session:

- Write two pages on your health and body.

Your Sexual Identity

OBJECTIVES

Discuss reasons to stick to facts in writing autobiography

Identify subjective influences on interpreting a life

Emphasize that interpretation of one's life should come from within, not from other members of the group

Explore the beneficial role of humor

Introduce theme 6: Your sexual identity

Share on theme 5: Your health and body

MATERIALS

Enrollment List

Flip chart or board and writing instrument

Plain white paper and pencils or crayons

Handout (Appendix B):

Theme 6: Your Sexual Identity

---

1. Get feedback on last week's writing assignment

Discuss with the large group any problems or insights arising from the writing assignment.

2. Distinguish between writing an autobiography and interpreting it

Facts are timeless, but the interpretation of those facts can change over time. Share these examples with the group.

The ancient Celts recorded the seasons and the movement of the sun with great accuracy, but their abstractions and interpretation of the causes of these events were inaccurate.

An adolescent boy regularly cut class to go surfing. The days were gorgeous, the surf was great, and when he was out there on a wave, nobody bugged him. His interpretation of his behavior might have been, "Teachers and school are stupid." At fifty, looking back on his youth, this individual might offer some other interpretation, such as "I couldn't pay attention in math. I hated it so much I just couldn't face it every day." The facts remain the same, but the man's interpretation of those facts has not stayed the same.

Encourage participants to stick to the concrete details of their lives when they write. What happened? What did the people around them do in a given situation? What do they remember about the sights, sounds, smells, and other details? How did they feel? Their interpretations of the meaning of these events may have changed over time.

As we get new information and mature, we tend to view events through a different lens; the lens changes shape with the accumulation of more life experience. Sticking to the facts as we write our autobiographies gives us the freedom to adapt and upgrade our interpretation of events as needed.

Participants can share their interpretation of their life events in small-group discussions. Remind everyone that in guided autobiography, participants should refrain from offering interpretation of *other* people's lives. There are several reasons for this.

a. Each life is unique

Even children in the same family experience a different phase in the family's development. Position in the family, temperament, and personality influence the way in which any child experiences life within the family and in the world outside.

b. The same events can have different effects

The Great Depression had a different impact in rural and urban areas. The experience of World War II was different for an infantry soldier, an officer in a training camp, a pilot, a worker in a defense plant, and the women and families left to hold down the fort at home. A general once said that in times of war, he knew when to be afraid and when to wait. His wife didn't know, so she was afraid all the time. Perspective has an impact on how one experiences events. Age at the time of an event makes a difference, too.

c. The context of events differs
Being in a car accident is different from witnessing one. A move that divides a family is different from a move that a family makes together. The general state of your life and your family situation when a particular event occurs may influence how you respond to it.

d. There is more than one way to view life
Writing about the facts of our lives, and adding whatever personal interpretations or insights we wish to share with the group, stimulates others to look at their own lives in new ways. As the contrast among people's personal interpretations of life events makes clear, life presents infinite variety in the way we experience it and the way we interpret our experiences. There is no one right way.

3. Discuss the beneficial role of humor in life and life review
Humor is a very effective tool for relieving tension and making difficult memories easier to remember, write, and share. Humor typically plays on some kind of universal experience or desire and, with a twist, helps us see the experience or desire in a new way. Humor is often biting, but it can also be compassionate, help our understanding, and provide a sense of common ground.

In our guided autobiography workshops, in the first, introductory session, we often offer a humorous definition of autobiography:

Autobiography is the story of your best friend written by your worst enemy.

This definition addresses the ambiguous feelings people normally have as they begin to write their memoirs. Confronting the feelings with humor helps us relax and brings the idea of writing a life history down to earth. The quip makes participants feel they are on an equal footing. We aren't always our worst enemy, but we all know that sometimes we can be. Humor reduces the size and the power of the enemy.

Encourage participants to use humor in their writing if they feel comfortable doing so. Humor can reduce any despicable enemy into something small and funny. The terrible schoolteacher of the past or the demon drill sergeant can be recalled in detail but experienced with a smile or a laugh if a joke can take the sting out of the memory.

Humor can ease tension in large- and small-group discussions, too, as long as the humor is not used at someone else's expense. Many of the life themes explored in guided autobiography generate discussion of sensitive topics among people with quite different outlooks on life. For example, group members may have quite different attitudes about politics or religion and even about many aspects of daily living, such as sex, smoking, or modes of dress. Guided autobiography should foster an atmosphere that encourages all participants to tell the stories of their lives in an honest, relaxed, and inoffensive manner. Appropriate use of humor facilitates this.

Whether an anecdote or a one-liner, humor usually comes from an unexpected association or twist in perspective. Here are some examples:

- Play on words: "He had his whole future behind him."
- Exaggeration: "My grandfather was so big he was on both sides of the family tree."
- Creating a funny image: Woody Allen said, "I don't like L.A. I don't get mellow. I ripen and rot."

The goal of a guided autobiography workshop is to help participants tell their life histories in plain, everyday language. Recounting their stories with humor may help people be more accepting of their lives as they are or have been. Tell participants not to stress or strain over the issue of humor, but encourage them to seek opportunities to incorporate humor into their lives, their group discussions, and their writing.

While on the topic of humor, share this thought:

> *Those who laugh . . . last.*
> —Stacy Lynn Skinner

4. Introduce theme 6: Your sexual identity

The title of this theme may raise eyebrows and anxiety among some participants. Occasionally groups request that men and women meet separately for sharing on this theme. However, as the sensitizing questions indicate, this theme covers much more than physical sexuality. Involving both men and women in a discussion of this topic can be very helpful and enlightening. Remind participants that they themselves choose what material they want to share.

In the past thirty years, the roles of men and women have changed dramatically. Engage participants in discussion around the following questions. Brainstorm together and be sensitive to your group. Allow other lines of discussion to substitute for these if they seem more appropriate.

a. Role models
What role models and relationships influenced you as you developed your sexual identity? Movie stars, heroes in books, parents, relatives, friends, and siblings all may influence how we view our roles as men or women and what we view as the ideal man or woman. How have your ideas changed as you have grown up and grown older?

b. Cultural factors
How have the following affected men and women and their relationships with each other?

- Feminism
- Women joining the workforce
- The sexual revolution
- Changing concepts of the "ideal" man or woman
- Pop culture
- Cultural diversity

How did stereotypes affect your self-image and your goals as a man or a woman? The feminist movement challenged our way of raising girls and fought to break down stereotypes that it saw as hampering the development of girls and women. An emerging collection of literature is now looking at male stereotypes and examining how we can do a better job of raising boys to become exceptional men. We always seem to be seeking a balance.

What conflicts do immigrants encounter while raising their children in a culture that may have different sexual mores or different role expectations for men and women? Ask participants if they have had experience in another culture that has influenced their personal views about sex or body image.

c. Age

How does aging affect the way we think about physical beauty, sexuality, and expectations for relationships? What are the characteristics of a mature man or woman? Consider the following situation. Before age discrimination was a litigious issue, a classified ad ran in a newspaper asking for a "mature woman to serve as a liaison between professional services providers and low-income families." What characteristics do you think the employer was seeking? Contrast these to the characteristics of a young woman. How would the employer have to word the ad today to get a person with the desired characteristics? What are the characteristics of a mature man? Of a young man?

Imagine someone you respect describing you as a mature man or a mature woman. What characteristics would you like ascribed to you? Do these characteristics describe you now? Can they be developed?

What is the impact of living to be eighty or ninety instead of forty-five (as at the beginning of the twentieth century) on sexual roles and expectations in love relationships?

5. Hand out the theme sheets and go over the sensitizing questions

As you go over the sensitizing questions with the group, provide examples from your own life, where appropriate, and invite group members to add their stories. Here are examples from previous workshops.

> *When I was about nine, my mother gave me a book called* Where Do Babies Come From? *It had been carefully saved since my brother had used it twelve years earlier. I read the book and asked a few questions. Then I was on my own until the night before my wedding when my mother passed on the wisdom passed down from her mother and grandmother: "Never say* no *to your husband in the bedroom." Perhaps she wanted to add something more, but all she said was, "and never put bananas in the refrigerator." This was an embarrassing moment for both of us, but at twenty, I thought I knew more about everything than she did, so her advice really didn't matter to me.*

I remember the atmosphere at school being somewhat sexualized. Sex seemed to be the only topic of conversation. Everyone told huge lies about sex. Girls came in by bus every six weeks for a dance. We loved those slow dances. We knew which girls would let you dance too close for propriety and not squeal on you later. Our favorite trick to avoid trouble was to make lots of swirls and press in close when your partner needed support. The big rule was never let a girl feel an erection while you danced with her. If accused of this, the rumor was that you would be immediately kicked out of school without a hearing.

I grew up in a neighborhood with about twenty boys and three girls. I wasn't really a tomboy, but playing with the boys was definitely where the action was. We played war and cops and robbers together all the time until I was about nine. Then the boys entered a "no girls allowed" phase. We girls filled empty sample bottles of Avon perfume with colored water and put them in an empty sewing basket and borrowed a stethoscope and other equipment from my little brother's doctor kit, then presented our plan to the boys. We were the nurses and would treat them on the battlefield. Once they died, they could come alive and rejoin the battle only after receiving medical treatment. (Naturally, we triaged the ones who were nice to us first. The others had to wait a long time for treatment before they could rejoin the battle.) The boys liked the idea, so at least for another summer, the boys and girls played together, but clearly the sexual roles were evolving.

I can remember being a reasonably attractive adolescent but very shy. I went to dances and stood with my friends praying for some cute boy to come and ask me to dance. Then, when someone looked at me, I would pray that he wouldn't come over and used every ounce of body language and negative energy I could to ward him away. What an awful time! I would have loved having a male friend I could really talk to, but I wouldn't risk getting close.

6. Ask people to draw a picture of themselves as adolescents

If time permits before the break, ask group participants to take ten minutes to draw a picture of themselves as adolescents. What did they wear? What did they say? (They can use "balloons" to indicate this.) Ask them to write down the names of people whom they wanted to be like. If they could speak now with the adolescent they once were, what would they say? What advice would they give? The group should take a few minutes to divide into pairs and share on this topic.

7. Take a ten-minute break

8. Reassemble the small groups for sharing stories
In the small groups, participants share on theme 5: your health and body.

9. Recap the tasks to complete before the next session
Instruct participants to accomplish the following task for the next session:

- Write two pages on your sexual identity.

Your Experiences with and Ideas about Death

OBJECTIVES
Discuss the role of confidant relationships
Introduce theme 7: Your experiences with and ideas about death
Share on theme 6: Your sexual identity

MATERIALS
Enrollment List
Flip chart or board and writing instrument
Handout (Appendix B):
   Theme 7: Your Experiences with and Ideas about Death

---

1. Get feedback on last week's writing assignment

Ask members of the large group whether they have any questions, comments, or insights on sexual identity.

2. Review the role of confidant relationships

Confidants, support groups, and networks of friends and business associates help reduce stress and help us achieve balance in our lives. We can absorb sources of stress, such as divorce, death, a move, serious illness, unemployment, or retirement, more easily when we have empathy and encouragement from other human beings. Confidant relationships help us regain a sense of equilibrium and optimism about the future. A supportive network, including a guided autobiography group, can be very powerful in helping us find our strengths and achieve more balance in our lives. Someone once said, "Life hardens what is soft in us and softens what is hard." Confidants can help in mending the wounds life inflicts and restoring a more balanced perspective. The joys of life become sweeter when shared with others.

Confidant relationships may be difficult to develop and maintain in our fast-paced society. As in guided autobiography groups, developing the trust necessary for a confidant relationship requires time. Ask participants to share their experiences with confidant relationships.

- Where have you found confidants?
- How have confidant relationships helped you?
- Where would you look for confidants if you felt a need for them?

Most of us have only a few confidants during our lives. Many people find themselves without a confidant at times of greatest need. Churches, grief ministries, support groups, parenting classes, and various other resources offer support, perspective, and care similar to that which a confidant relationship can provide. These groups sometimes bring people together who remain friends after the crisis has passed. At the end of a guided autobiography workshop, many participants say that one of their goals is to devote more time to nurturing relationships.

Being a good listener and encourager is the other side of a confidant relationship. One gives as well as receives.

3. Introduce theme 7: Your experiences with and ideas about death

Death is part of life. It is something every living thing must face. But the fact of death is difficult to grasp. Most of us have experienced the death of relatives or friends. The early death of a parent or other loved one can put an indelible stamp on someone's life. The importance of death, its ubiquity, its mystery, and the pain people may have before death, make it a sensitive matter to discuss.

Begin by asking group members for their earliest experiences with death. Perhaps it was the death of a pet. Ask if, as children, they performed rituals around the burial of a pet. Share your own experiences. One workshop participant shared the following story.

When my daughter was four, she won a goldfish at a community fair. Months later, the fish died. When we asked our daughter what she wanted to do with it, she tearfully asked our advice. We suggested burying the fish in the garden or flushing him down the toilet. The toilet would lead the fish eventually back to the sea, we said. So Tamara chose flushing it down the toilet. We gathered around the toilet, and Tamara dropped in the fish and flushed. As the fish whirled down, Tamara shouted, "I changed my mind!"

I think she felt that dual instinct of wanting life back and wanting to know what happened to her friend, the fish, after death.

Point out that of all life themes, this theme on experiences with and ideas about death is likely to reveal the strongest and most varied array of religious, philosophical, familial, and individual attitudes, emotions, and rituals. Tell participants to write about their own experiences with and feelings about death. Every point of view warrants respect because it is a true reflection of each individual's history. Unless a church group sponsors your workshop, participants' beliefs may range from agnostic or atheist to devout belief in a formal religion. Some group members may believe firmly in life after death, while others may be just as certain that there is no such thing. Many participants may be struggling with ambiguous feelings somewhere between these two positions. Emphasize yet again that the point of group discussion is not to judge what is right or wrong but to encourage people to write down their own histories and to learn from the stories of others. Actually, the contrast of beliefs often helps individuals understand their own attitudes and beliefs better so they can do a better job of writing their autobiographies.

As a leader, be sensitive to your group. Frequently, the younger members of a group have the most difficulty discussing death. If they are still focused on developing their own sense of identity and accomplishments, the thought of death may feel like a threat to their goals and aspirations. Older participants may be more pragmatic in accepting their mortality; they may be concerned more with the process of dying than with the state of death. An older participant in one of our workshops wrote, "When it is my time to go, I want to go with dignity, quickly and with no pain."

A leader who is uneasy or reluctant about discussing death will project tentativeness to the group and probably will not be able to encourage open discussion of issues related to death. It is helpful if you prepare for this session by reading contemporary literature that reflects a drift toward open discussion of such topics as assisted suicide, euthanasia, and hospice care because these issues are quite likely to be mentioned by participants.

Funeral rites are a relatively unthreatening and interesting gateway to discussing experiences with death, especially in groups with a variety of ethnic and religious perspectives. Ask participants whether they have attended a funeral in a culture different from their own. What did they learn? What was their reaction? This can lead to a discussion of the impact of death as experienced by members of the group.

In introducing the topic of death, keep in mind that your goal is to help participants in recalling their significant experiences with death and organizing their thoughts about how their views were shaped, not to support a particular philosophy or social point of view.

4. Ask participants what sorts of things influence our attitudes toward death

Brainstorm with the group on factors that influence attitudes toward death. Some examples:

- Age
- Changes in life circumstances
- Changes in relationships with siblings
- Writing autobiography
- Hospice programs
- Role models
- Cultural influences
- Religious beliefs

Perceived nearness to the end of life affects our perspective on death, and our views on death may change as our life circumstances change. As we age, we may tend to reflect on our memories and rearrange them in a different order or give them different weight than we would under other circumstances or at a different stage of life. Sibling relationships tend to become more important later in life, for example, and they can help us reconcile unresolved issues from childhood. This process can affect our attitudes toward death.

Autobiography tends to help us accept life as it has been lived. It helps us put aside anger and the need to block or suppress memories.

Hospice programs often give families a rich time of reconciliation and acceptance during a terminal illness. Ask whether any group members have had such an experience.

Everyone struggles with how to achieve a peaceful acceptance of mortality while still remaining fully engaged in life. Ask participants about people who have been role models for them.

Cultural differences influence people's attitudes toward death. In many cultures death is viewed as part of life, not just the end of a life. In Madagascar, people worship their ancestors and believe in a union of family members, deceased, living, and yet to be born. They open tombs and bring out the remains of their dead to join the living for a special feast day. In Mexico, November 1, the Day of the Dead, is one of the most important days of the year. Families take flowers and the favorite foods of their deceased loved ones to the graveyard, and the atmosphere is very festive. In some cultures, following a death, the women come together to wail loudly for a prescribed number of days; in others, the response is to keep a stiff upper lip and to carry on, almost as if nothing important had happened. Ask group members what sorts of cultural influences have shaped their attitudes toward death.

Religious beliefs have a profound impact on attitudes toward death. If one believes in life after death, death is regarded as a passage.

5. Hand out the theme sheet and go over the sensitizing questions
Go over the sensitizing questions for this session's theme, sharing your own experiences and inviting discussion from members of the large group. Here are examples from past workshops.

When my mother died, it was a great relief. I feel awfully guilty saying that, but she was a really awful person. She was an alcoholic, crabby and demanding as heck. All my life, I felt more like her mother. It was a hard job I was glad to give up!

I come from a large, multigeneration family, and death has been a part of life for me for as long as I can remember. The first funeral I can remember was for a great aunt who died when she was in her eighties. I was three or four. The luncheon after the funeral was a great time for cousins to play together, and there was a lot of warm chatter among adult family members. There were tears, but they were interspersed with laughter and fun memories. I remember people saying, "She will be so happy in heaven with Uncle Pat (her husband) and her sisters. They are probably playing bridge right now." So I thought heaven was just a party I wasn't old enough to attend yet. I had no fear of my own death until I had children. That fear stems from a sense of responsibility for them.

My younger brother died at the age of fifty-three when he was struck from behind while riding his bicycle home from a bar near his rented mobile home. I heard about it from his estranged girlfriend, Doris. Doris and Jack were in the process of reconciliation, but she had recently kicked him out again because of his unchecked drinking. The drinking had cost him his job, too. The funeral was held near Mom's home and was hosted for free by the local church. If it had taken place in Jack's hometown, we could have held it in the back of a van. Most of our family and more than fifty of Mom's friends showed up. The minister mentioned God's mercy and love and Jack's resting peacefully in heaven. That set me back because the thought of Jack's being in heaven never crossed my mind. I personally don't believe in the hereafter, but maybe Jack is in heaven. Who am I to determine something like that? I hope for his sake that he is.

My death of choice would be painless and peaceful, not tormented by a series of futile, pointless hospital treatments. On November 27, 1996, the doctor told me, "The cancer was much larger than we anticipated. I can only hazard a guess that we bought three years. Naturally, we hope for more for you." Last July [1999], the same doctor said, "Frankly, I am surprised you are still alive." If the cancer returns, I will not seek alternative medicines but will opt for a clean death. I have requested in my will that I be cremated and my ashes scattered over the ocean, not from a boat but from a plane. Guess what? At last I will get my boyhood wish to fly, and all on my own—solo.

Everything I need to know about death, I learned from my father. Just two weeks after his seventy-third birthday, my mother had a stroke, and we were struggling to keep her home. Dad said he didn't feel well. He was wheezing, and I thought he had the flu. When I took him to the doctor, we discovered he had had a heart attack. While he was recovering in the hospital critical care unit, I received a call from the doctor saying that X-rays taken to assess heart damage revealed that he had a tumor in his right lung. The biopsy showed cancer had spread to Dad's lymph nodes. *He had nine to twelve months to live. For several weeks, Dad lived in denial. The nurses at the hospital suggested I read Elisabeth Kubler-Ross's book* On Death and Dying. *It became my guide to my father's final journey. To give Dad the dignity he deserved, I wanted the process to be in his control as much as possible. I miss my father every day. He was a wonderful husband, father, and grandfather. I try to remember more than the dignity he achieved despite the pain and suffering of his final months. I try also to celebrate his life and the impact his love had on his family and students. I think that is as close as one gets to immortality—to live on in the memories of those who remember you with love.*

6. Take a ten-minute break

7. Reassemble the small groups for sharing stories
In small groups, participants share their stories on theme 6: your sexual identity.

8. Recap the tasks to complete before the next session
Instruct participants to accomplish the following task for the next session:

- Write two pages on your experiences with and ideas about death.

Your Spiritual Life and Values

OBJECTIVES

Clarify what group members mean by the word *spiritual*

Introduce theme 8: Your spiritual life and values

Share on theme 7: Your experiences with and ideas about death

MATERIALS

Enrollment List

Flip chart or board and writing instrument

Handouts (Appendix B):

Where to Go from Here?

Theme 8: Your Spiritual Life and Values

---

1. Get feedback on last week's writing assignment

Ask participants how the writing went last week. Was death an easy or difficult topic? Did thinking about it and writing about it have any impact on their attitudes toward death?

2. Introduce theme 8: Your spiritual life and values

a. Spirituality *has a variety of meanings*

Ask participants what the word *spiritual* means to them. Thinking about or discussing spiritual matters may at first be uncomfortable for group members who are atheist or agnostic or who have had negative experiences with religion. Explain to everyone that in guided autobiography, we use the word *spiritual* in the most general sense, and participants can apply secular or religious interpretations—whatever seems most appropriate in recording their personal histories. We all have a spiritual element in our nature, regardless of our religious beliefs. Some have defined it as the part of us that searches for truth, values, and meaning in our lives. The history of our spiritual life may include experiences with nature and with people that have contributed to the development of the part of ourselves that cannot be defined in physical terms.

The *Oxford English Dictionary* defines *spirit* as "the animating or vital principle in humans and animals; that which gives life to the organism in contrast to its purely material elements; the breath of life." Poet Dylan Thomas described spirit in this way: "The force that through the green fuse drives the flower / Drives my green age."

A history of one's spiritual life might include something about the restlessness many of us feel at one time or another as we attempt to find out who we are and what life means. The drive to understand this part of our humanity is shared by atheists, agnostics, and the devout of all the world's religions.

b. The quest for meaning and truth begins in early childhood

Ask participants what kinds of values and ethics their families taught them as children. Give examples from your own life. Here are some examples from previous workshops.

> *Whenever we argued as children, our mother would ask each of us how we thought the other fellow felt. It made us step out and put ourselves in the other person's shoes. Usually, after we all felt heard, the tension had dissipated and we went on with our play.*

> *We went to Sunday school every Sunday. My mother dropped us off and picked us up later. She only went to church on the holidays. I think she just liked this time to read the Sunday newspaper in peace.*

> *I can remember Dad saying so many times, "If you can't say something nice about someone, don't say it at all." Sometimes I would be bursting to tell about something someone else had done, but Dad was never interested in hearing about it.*

Use the following questions to stimulate participants' thinking or discussion on childhood influences on spirituality:

- Did the adults in your life practice what they preached?
- Did your family attend church?
- Did they discuss spiritual or moral values outside church?
- From their actions, what did you sense that they valued most in life?
- What kinds of early experiences made you feel special or unique or aware that there was some part of you that could not be described in physical terms?

Our earliest spiritual experiences usually fall into the realm of feelings and emotions rather than thought. Ask participants whether they remember any early experiences of well-being, peace, or acceptance. Here is an example.

My father was sole owner of a small business and worked very long hours six or seven days a week. We rarely took even weekend vacations, but one year, he closed down his business for a week. I climbed into the back of our 1952 Chevy sedan with my brother and little sister. Mom sat at Dad's side in the front seat, and we headed west for Wyoming to spend several days in the mountains with a childhood friend of Mother's. Her friend had a stone cabin in the mountains beside a trout stream.

In those days, the mountain streams ran so clear and clean that we could drink from them. A split-rail fence ran from the cabin around twenty acres of national forest land with trails, beaver ponds, a network of trout streams, and meadows. The lodge-pole pine forest was home to white-tailed deer and elk, including a buck with a magnificent rack. My older brother and I (I was six, and he was seven) had free run of the property as long as we didn't cross the fence. We could always, the adults explained, walk until we came to the fence and follow it back to the cabin. Sleeping in the cabin at night with moonlight casting shadows on the stuffed animals and hunting trophies in the great room was a bit spooky, but I was always so tired from the day's adventures that I quickly fell too soundly asleep to worry. The real spiritual experience came in the mornings. First light streamed through the picture window onto the daybed where I slept. Every day, as reliable as clockwork, I awoke to see a doe and her two fawns drinking from the stream gurgling gently just outside the window.

I was too young to put words to it then, but I was aware of feeling so safe, small but important. All the wonders of this place were a gift. The things I loved about those mornings are things I have loved ever since—waking at dawn, enjoying the early light and quiet while others still sleep, the sense of adventure and freedom I shared with my brother, the lure of the mountains, love of nature, and love of tall tales told around a fire. Also, I think, at the heart of all this feeling of well-being was a sense that I owed that very special week to the deep and enduring friendship of my mother and her friend. That was something I wanted in my life, too.

c. Adolescence is often a time of questioning or rebellion

Each of us must develop our own system of values. Questioning helps us do this. We examine the values taught to us by our families and by society and decide which ones we accept and which we reject. This is a normal part of growing up. Periods of questioning and rebellion may occur throughout life. They are a natural part of spiritual growth and development. Times of questioning often are followed by a return to faith or beliefs with a more personal and meaningful commitment.

Adolescence often brings on the first period of questioning or rebellion. We flex our spiritual muscles and our minds to find out who we are. Teenagers often seem to be engaged in battle with issues of spirit, as if this battle will give them a better understanding of their place in the universe.

In the large group, ask participants to ponder and discuss the following questions:

- When you were a teenager, what kinds of experiences helped you find out who you were? Did you ever have to defend something you believed in? Did disappointment in other people's actions help define your values?
- How old were you when you developed your own sense of personal values? What ideas did you reject? What values did you embrace as your own?
- Was your family religious?

d. Mentors and role models can influence our spiritual journeys

Ask participants what role models or mentors have influenced their spiritual journeys. There is an expression "Life never gives us more than we can handle," but another expression says "Life always gives us more than we can handle; that is why we have each other."

Americans revere the idea of rugged individualism, but interdependence can be a positive concept, too. Encourage participants to think about the role of mentors.

- Who has helped you along the way?
- What roles have mentors played in the evolution of your beliefs, values, and ethics? How have they taught you to be more true to yourself and be more than you thought you could be?
- Have you been a mentor to others? How has mentoring others helped you on your own life journey?

3. Ask participants to draw a visual map of their spiritual journey

Encourage participants, before they write their two pages for next session, to make a map of their spiritual journey. Ask them what images they could use to illustrate their paths. Brainstorm together on this topic, noting ideas on the board or flip chart. Metaphors such as thunderstorms, lightning, sunshine, rainbows, earthquakes of trouble or illness, ascents to mountain peaks of understanding or accomplishment, rocky canyons of despair, burned bridges, deadly curves, placid lakes, peaceful valleys, personal or professional battlefields, or hearts and flowers might be useful. Encourage participants to use a big piece of white paper and to have fun. Tell them to be free in their drawing. Their writing should be easier after this exercise. Suggest that they bring their maps to the next session to share in their small groups.

4. Hand out the theme sheet and go over the sensitizing questions

Go over the sensitizing questions for this theme, giving examples from your own life and encouraging participation from the group. Here are examples from previous workshops.

I have abused my body. When I was about fifty, I started menopause and began to gain weight. At first it was only ten pounds. Then I would diet to lose ten pounds and gain fifteen back. I never got obese, but when my husband filed for divorce, I became obsessed with food. I ate and drank to mask my unhappiness. It was the most awful time of my life. During those years, I gained and lost a great deal of weight, bouncing from one fad diet to the next until, finally, nothing worked. The only thing I lost was my self-confidence. I weighed two hundred pounds. Then, through the grace of God, I found a twelve-step program. That was five years ago. I found the inner strength and spirituality I had lost. The program helped me recover from a terrible divorce, the estrangement of my family, and the closing of my business. Most of all, it helped me regain my health and self-confidence. I have never been happier than I am today.

My primary experience with God as a child was through nature. We lived next to "the woods," an undeveloped part of our suburban neighborhood. I liked to find secret hiding places, beautiful spots where I would sit and feel peaceful, almost like meditating. I remember one spot where violets bloomed. I loved being by myself exploring natural places. Of course, I ended up with a lot of poison ivy, but it did give me a feeling of being part of God's creation.

When I was in high school, I was part of a church youth group. The Civil Rights movement was starting, and I was quite concerned about that. We'd sometimes have black students come to our meeting. I argued with my parents about this. They talked about how property values would drop if blacks moved into our white neighborhood, and I was very disturbed by that. The youth group experience made me aware of the social issues of the day, but I am not sure what I learned about Christianity. It has taken me all my adult life to figure out what Christianity is all about.

I can't remember getting much of anything out of attending services. When I was in high school, I daydreamed and sometimes wrote poetry during services. I liked the stories associated with the holidays, but I don't think I had a sense of how they might influence my own faith.

5. Ask participants to think about where they want to go from here

Distribute the handout "Where to Go from Here?" Ask participants to spend time before the next session thinking about how they would like to pursue their autobiographies after the workshop has ended. By this time, participants have done a lot of writing and tapped into a wealth of memories. As the workshop nears its end, people may be beginning to ask themselves, "Where do I go from here?" They may want to continue with group work or figure out a way to refine and focus their autobiographies into finished projects. Tell them to let you know what additional guidance or support they need to move forward. Ask them to write a paragraph or more at home explaining what they would like to do with their work and asking any questions they would like you to address in the final session. They should hand in the paper at the beginning of the next session.

6. Take a ten-minute break

7. Reassemble in small groups for sharing stories
In their small groups, participants share on theme 7: your experiences with and ideas about death.

8. Recap the tasks to complete before the next session
Instruct participants to accomplish the following tasks for the next session:

- Draw a road map of your spiritual life.
- Write down your ideas and questions about where you want to go from here with your autobiography.
- Write two pages on your spiritual life and values.

SESSION 9

Your Goals and Aspirations

OBJECTIVES

Get written feedback from participants on plans for their
autobiographies after the workshop

Confirm names, addresses, phone and fax numbers, and e-mail
addresses for a roster

Discuss the concept of a balanced life portfolio

Introduce theme 9: Your goals and aspirations

Turn participants' attention to goals for the future

Make plans for the final session

Share on theme 8: Your spiritual life and values

MATERIALS

Enrollment List

Flip chart or board and writing instrument

Handouts (Appendix B):

   Your Life Portfolio

   Leader's Life Portfolio, or Sample Life Portfolio in Appendix B

   Abilities, Opportunities, and Responsibilities

   Theme 9: Your Goals and Aspirations

   Evaluation Form

---

1. Get feedback on last week's writing assignment

Ask participants whether they have any problems to discuss or special in-
sights to share. How did they get on with mapping their spiritual journeys?
How well did this diversion to visual instead of written expression work?
Some people will like it more than others.

We take in about 80 percent of the information we receive through sight. Instead of taking photographs when he traveled, modernist architect Richard Neutra made quickly executed drawings and watercolors. He found that the time and concentration required for these tasks created a more lasting, more integrated memory. Ask group members whether the visual exercise of mapping triggered more unexpected memories or new associations.

2. Collect completed "Where to Go from Here?" handouts

Use the information and questions participants have submitted on the "Where to Go from Here?" sheets to prepare and guide discussion for the final session. Invite group members to bring in books, scrapbooks, collages, artwork, or anything else that might give their fellow participants ideas about how to present their work. A portion of the last session will be devoted to "think tank" time about book titles, resources, and other information.

If some group members have not prepared comments or questions at home, ask them to do so during the break so they can give you their feedback before they leave the session today.

3. Collect information for a roster of participants

Ask if anyone objects to having his or her name, address, phone number, fax number, or e-mail address on a roster to be distributed to members of the workshop. Explain that you will create the roster from the information forms or cards filled out in the first session. Ask anyone who needs to update this information or who does not want to be included in the roster to let you know in a written note, which should be handed in now.

Some groups want to continue meeting informally, and most enjoy periodic reunions; the roster helps with ongoing communication. Bring up this topic with participants now. If a group wants to continue to meet, the group members should designate someone to organize the first reunion, or the workshop leader (for whole-group reunions) or small-group facilitators can agree to take on that job.

4. Introduce the idea of a balanced life portfolio

Leading a satisfying life involves finding balance in the trilogy of life—work, play, and love. People under high stress have trouble establishing a good balance between these elements, and this imbalance perpetuates stress.

The balance is rarely perfect or permanent, but, like acrobats, we constantly must make adjustments to try to achieve equilibrium. When we lean too far in one direction, we can sense that we are in trouble and that other important aspects of our lives need more attention. Ask participants how they sense that their lives are out of balance.

- Do you feel the imbalance, or do you realize it through cues from other people?
- What steps do you take to correct the imbalance? Do you use the old tried and true coping skills—denial, repression, fantasy, and humor—to get through stressful periods, or do you make substantive changes to reduce stress?
- Why is it sometimes so hard to make lifestyle choices that would support a more balanced life?

5. Discuss the benefits of a balanced life portfolio

A balanced life portfolio enables us to handle change and respond to the unexpected challenges life sometimes throws at us. Putting all our eggs in one basket is a bad idea in investments, and it is a bad idea in life. It can make us less resilient to change and to trauma. Men traditionally have held more specialized roles in life than women. They tend to focus strongly on their careers, define themselves through their work, and show their love for their families through their roles as providers. In other words, they tend to keep all their eggs in one basket. Men who have invested most of their life energy in work usually have to do more adjusting to retirement than do men who have developed hobbies and networks of friends outside work or have been involved in community work.

Women tend to hold more diversified life portfolios. The empty-nest syndrome can be difficult for women who have defined themselves almost solely as mothers. However, even if a woman's primary occupation has been staying at home to raise children, *motherhood* is an umbrella for many other roles. Mothers are de facto teachers, nurses, transmitters of values, chauffeurs, community volunteers, event planners, contractors for services, counselors, social secretaries, and more. Today, the majority of women also do work outside their homes, but their diversified roles continue—they are just taking their multitasking capabilities into another arena. With the ability to focus on many things at once, they have many interests and skills that can carry them forward, even when one of their key roles changes or is no longer appropriate. Nonetheless, the challenge of balancing the trilogy of work, play, and love is difficult.

At the beginning of the twenty-first century, the roles of both men and women are less rigidly defined than in the past. Finding enough time to do everything on our agenda is a major problem for most of us. Roles expand, but there are still only twenty-four hours in a day. The choices we make about how we spend those twenty-four hours help define who we are and what our priorities are. Often we dream of making changes, but we are so focused on the demands of each day that the months and years can pass before we wake up to the fact that "as we spend our days, so we spend our lives."

Tell the group that they are going to take a look at their life portfolios to see how balanced they are and how they might be able to redirect their energy and time to achieve more balance.

6. Group exercise: Graphing a life portfolio

Purpose: To encourage participants to examine how past, present, and future goals affect their sense of balance in life.

Distribute "Your Life Portfolio" and be prepared to share your own life portfolio, which you have drawn up before the session (Appendix B contains an example). Describe how you distribute your time and why you use your time this way, where you see imbalances, and your goals for the future.

Ask participants to consider the question, "How balanced is my life portfolio?" Rarely does one come to the end of life and say, "I wish I had worked more," but there might be exceptions. A woman who has stayed home raising children for many years may have latent career ambitions she wants to pursue when the children become more independent. A man who has recently retired from a demanding career may want to have a second career or to pursue leisure activities or involvement in public service.

Go over the instructions at the top of the handout with the large group. Ask participants to take about ten minutes to graph their life portfolios as they now are and (with another color or a dotted line) as they would like them to be in the future. They can then share their portfolio with a partner.

As a large group, discuss the difficulties many couples have at retirement and the reasons why a diverse portfolio is good if health declines, a job suddenly disappears, or you lose a spouse or partner. Discuss the fact that one usually must give something up to make room for change and for renewal in life. This is one reason why transitions can be so uncomfortable.

7. Introduce theme 9: Your goals and aspirations

Until now, the explorations of life themes in the workshop have taken participants' attention back to early childhood and brought them forward to the present. The theme for the final session, goals and aspirations, also goes back into personal history, but it also invites group members to think ahead by considering their goals and aspirations for the future.

Yoga teachers tell their students, "Honor the past, take responsibility for the future, but live and act fully in the present." This is good advice. It puts our lives in context. The final theme of this workshop helps create a bridge between our past histories and our goals and aspirations for the future.

By this time, participants will have gained new insight about how events have shaped them and how their personalities and personal choices have shaped their lives. Most of them will have gained appreciation for their own strengths and weaknesses. Examining and integrating life experiences through guided autobiography encourages people to honor their strengths and use them to accept or overcome their weaknesses. Many participants will have rediscovered old interests and talents that they want to develop further. Ask participants, "How have your feelings about yourself and your life changed? What strengths have you discovered in your stories? What are your goals for the future?"

In session 4, participants wrote down the five characteristics they thought best described themselves and selected the single characteristic they found most fitting. Ask participants whether, during the course of the workshop, they have discovered new characteristics or rediscovered old ones they would like to add to their list. Ask them if they would pick a new, single characteristic as most descriptive of themselves or their life.

8. Hand out the theme sheet and go over the sensitizing questions

As you go over the sensitizing questions for this theme, give some examples from your own life and invite participants to do the same. Here are examples from past workshops.

When my husband died four years ago, I held a very unhappy view of the future. Like a lot of other women, I couldn't imagine how I could go on after losing my husband. I spent a lot of time trying to understand where I had been so that I would know where I could go. During those hard times, I discovered a lot about my interests. I came out of that period of soul-searching feeling that life had been pretty good to me. Since then, I have become more future-oriented. My main goal is to get a life other than work. While I want to continue to expand my career, I have dedicated myself to enhancing relationships, especially my relationship with my daughter. I want to enjoy the outdoors, return to spiritual pursuits, become more involved with the community, and become financially secure. I've also worked on improving the "package" I present to the world. I haven't gone "Hollywood" exactly, but I had been influenced by negative role models in the past. I realize that if I want to be healthy, energetic, secure, and have fun and be happy, I need to present that attitude to others.

In my early years, my goals were to be smart and popular. My goals came from my parents. They were models of smart, popular, attractive, and competent people. Later the feminist and hippie movements that concentrated on individual awareness influenced my personal goals. My goals and aspirations are now more inner-directed.

I was influenced by Eastern philosophy and became a psychologist. One of my goals was to have a good relationship with a man. That seemed like a simple goal. My parents have been married seventy years, and my mother always claimed her greatest accomplishment was keeping my father pleased. It wasn't so simple for me. I am an only child, and I felt it was important for my parents to know I would be there for them. Now my goals are to (1) be free, (2) live in the moment, (3) be connected to my highest self, (4) not get caught up in performing for others, (5) be amused, playful, and live with humor, (6) be joyful and let my gratitude inform my acts of creativity, and (7) be kind and forgiving toward myself and others.

At eighty, I suppose I could feel fulfilled and stop learning, but I still have goals:
1. I must still write my autobiography using poetry I have written through the years.
2. I must become computer savvy.
3. I should learn to play bridge again to become more social.
4. I want to participate more actively in my grandchildren's endeavors.

5. I must do everything possible to keep up my relatively good health. (I started an exercise class this week.)

9. Distribute the handout "Abilities, Opportunities, and Responsibilities"

Participants may like to take home the handout "Abilities, Opportunities, and Responsibilities" as another example of how one person who experienced guided autobiography articulated his goals for the future.

10. Ask participants to fill out the Evaluation Forms

Explain to the group the usefulness of getting feedback from workshop participants. Ask them to fill out the Evaluation Forms at home and return them in the final session.

11. Discuss plans for the final session

Food often sets a celebratory tone. A potluck dinner or a cake offered by the workshop leader or the sponsoring organization celebrates the friendships that have been formed and the discoveries each participant has made. Ask participants what sort of celebration they would like.

12. Ask small-group members to write good wishes for one another

Before the break, ask small-group facilitators to suggest to their group members that, during the next week, they write good wishes for each member of their small group to distribute at the final session.

At the end of several weeks of sharing personal histories, small-group participants usually feel strong bonds and wish one another the very best. Facilitators should ask participants to write a one-sentence message on a 3-inch × 5-inch card (or other small note stationery) for each member of their small group, expressing a wish or wishes for that person's future. The notes will be distributed at the final small-group session, and each person will read the wishes aloud after completing the reading of his or her paper.

13. Take a ten-minute break

14. Reassemble the small groups for sharing of stories

In small groups, participants share their writing on theme 8: your spiritual life and values.

15. Recap the tasks to complete before the next session
Instruct participants to accomplish the following tasks for the next session:

- Write two pages on your goals and aspirations.
- Write good wishes for each member of your small group.
- Fill out the Evaluation Form.

Wrapping It Up

OBJECTIVES

Discuss ideas for book and chapter titles in autobiography

Address concerns raised by participants who want to continue their autobiography projects

Collect the completed evaluation forms

Share on theme 9: Your goals and aspirations

Provide time for final thoughts and goodbyes in the large group

MATERIALS

Enrollment List

Flip chart or board and writing instrument

Handouts:

    Workshop roster

    Annotated Reading List (the back of this manual)

    Extra copies of Evaluation Form (Appendix B)

    Choosing a Title for the Story of Your Life (Appendix B)

    List of local resources for paper, printing, and bookbinding (if possible)

---

1. Distribute workshop rosters and reading lists

Distribute copies of the workshop roster and the reading list on group members' chairs, or leave them by the door for participants to pick up later.

2. Collect completed Evaluation Forms

Collect all completed Evaluation Forms and have extra forms available for participants who have forgotten theirs or were absent at the last session.

Write a note on the flip chart or board reminding participants to hand in the forms before the break.

3. Provide refreshments
Have an attractive place for a cake or other food and refreshments to celebrate the last session. Provide an extra ten minutes of free time at the beginning of the session for people to get their refreshments and chat before officially starting the session.

4. Welcome and congratulate participants
In welcoming people to this last session, recognize again that writing an autobiography takes courage. Not everyone wants to do it. Tell them how impressed you have been with the work they have done. It took courage to look at their lives, to try to make sense of them, to write about them, and *then* to share their stories with others—but look what happened when they did!

After working on autobiography, we usually realize we have done pretty well in our lives. All of us have lived through good and bad times, and we have lived to write about it! We are survivors. We are capable men and women with still more to give to and get from life. We have met interesting new people and learned from their life stories. Group members may even want to see one another again after the workshop is over. (If you have not yet distributed the roster, tell group members where to pick it up.)

Most participants probably feel that what they have covered in the workshop is just the tip of the iceberg of their lives. Assure them that they all have many more stories to tell, and now they have some guidelines to help organize these stories. They may also have found one or more themes or directions of growth in their lives that they had not thought much about before taking the workshop.

5. Get feedback on last week's writing assignment
Ask group members how the writing on goals and aspirations went. Do they have any problems or insights to share? What kinds of aspirations do participants have for the future? Do they feel confident about attaining them?

6. Encourage participants to think of a title for their life story

Ask participants to consider their life as a book. What title is appropriate for their autobiography? What has been the central theme of their life? Distribute the handout "Choosing the Title for the Story of Your Life."

Explain that the guided autobiography workshop uses the word *autobiography* because it means simply the story of one's life as narrated by oneself. The word contains no judgment or expectation. However, encourage participants to create more exciting or descriptive titles for their stories. The handout contains examples to help stimulate their thinking. Read these, or ask one or more group members to read them, to the large group.

Ask participants to write down as many phrases as they can think of that might describe their lives. This is a brainstorming session. Tell group members to write down every idea, then to pick the three they like most and create three titles. Ask them to write their ideas on the handout. Take examples and ask each person why she or he chose that title.

Now each participant has three possible working titles. They may think of more as they continue their work.

7. Ask participants to think of chapter titles for their book

Participants should now think of some chapter titles for their autobiography. If they go back to the life graph exercise they completed in session 1, they will see major branching points, or turning points, in the plots of their lives. The intervals between the turning points could be chapters with rising or falling action.

- What title would you give to each chapter?
- What is the theme of the chapter you are now living? What is a good title for this chapter?
- What would you like the next chapter to be?

Time will not permit a deep exploration of this subject, but this brief discussion will give participants material to think about in the future.

8. Discuss with participants where they want to go from here

Be sure to address specific questions and issues participants raised in their written feedback on "Where to Go from Here?" Engage the large group in sharing ideas. Share the books, scrapbooks, and other samples of autobiographical presentations that you and the participants have brought in. If you have been able to prepare a list of local resources for paper, printing, and bookbinding, distribute this now.

The following suggestions to present to the group are related to issues that most frequently come up in this final session.

a. Think of ways to stimulate more writing

Expand on the themes you have already explored briefly. Perhaps each could become a chapter in your autobiography. Consider illustrating chapters with photos, drawings, and anecdotes. Find topics for additional themes (this can be done by brainstorming in the large group). For example:

- Roads I have not taken
- My likes and dislikes
- My attitudes toward children and child-rearing
- My sense of adventure
- My major friendships
- Major societal events and how they have influenced my life (Depression, World War II, Vietnam War, 1960s' activism, feminist movement, etc.)

Look in libraries or bookstores for other people's autobiographies and related literature. Many books contain guiding questions, although most cover more superficial subjects than does guided autobiography. Also use the library or bookstore to explore various genres of writing to see which best suits you and your story—children's books, poetry, personal essays, journals, letters, recipe books, humor.

b. Investigate ways of presenting ideas

Here are some useful tools for creating an attractive presentation for a life history:

- Computerized layout programs
- Custom binding services
- Scrapbooks in which to enter writing, photos, and drawings (Many

large bookstores, craft stores, and community adult education programs offer classes in making scrapbooks.)
- Photo albums that can hold sheets of writing paper as well as photos
  (Some albums are works of art in themselves.)
- Artful bookbinding (Many books and classes are available on bookbinding.)
- Various types of paper (Look in the Yellow Pages or ask a good printer
  to find paper sources near you that sell acid-free paper for use in your
  printer. Acid-free paper does not yellow with age.)

Quick-print shops offer a variety of binding options and papers. Spiral binding with attractive paper stock and cover stock can make a handsome and
durable book. Consider using text weight paper for the pages and cover
stock for the front and back cover.

c. Continue sharing

Sharing in autobiography workshops, especially in the small groups, tends
to create strong bonds and very fertile ground for learning more about oneself and about life. Participants may feel reluctant to see the group experience end. Many small groups continue to meet informally after the official
end of a ten-week workshop. Here are some ideas previous participants have
found helpful for maintaining contact:

- Trade names, phone numbers, and addresses with other group members (or make sure you have this information on the workshop roster)
  and continue to meet weekly, monthly, or periodically.
- If getting together physically is impossible, e-mail might work. However, personal contact is much more satisfying.
- Form a new group and teach new people the guided autobiography
  technique. You will continue to discover new things about yourself.
  Think of contexts in which people might benefit from guided autobiography. Themes can be adapted for older-adult groups, church groups,
  peer-counseling training groups, rehabilitation centers, or prisons.
- Form a writing group or take writing classes to further develop the
  writing you have begun in this workshop.
- Encourage your friends to take a guided autobiography workshop.

- Organize people who want to develop a desktop publishing version of their autobiography.

d. Investigate the possibilities of publishing

The world of commercial publishing is highly competitive. Dr. Seuss got seventy-six rejection letters before his first children's book was published. Autobiography writers who want to publish need to be realistic, but of course, unless you try, you will never know what is possible. There are many excellent classes on writing for publication. Rewriting through several drafts is part of the process of polishing a manuscript enough to warrant the attention of an editor and publisher. Participants interested in publishing their stories through a commercial publisher will benefit from further writing courses.

Self-publishing is another option, and books are available on this topic as well.

9. Explain how the remaining time will be spent

Ask for the remaining workshop evaluations. Explain that after the break, group members will share in small groups then come together for goodbyes and any closing thoughts. Announce what time the small groups will return to the large group for closing. Allow fifteen or twenty minutes for the final large-group session.

10. Take a ten-minute break

11. Reassemble the small groups to share stories

In small groups, facilitators should allow a few minutes for participants to distribute their good wishes to other group members. Invite participants to read aloud their received wishes after reading their two pages on theme 9: your goals and aspirations.

12. Reassemble the large group for sharing and some closing thoughts

In the large group, allow twenty minutes for group members to express what the guided autobiography experience has meant to them and what they would like to do next.

Tell participants you would like to share a few final thoughts, some quotations that may reflect ideas that have become clearer to them as they have written and shared their personal histories and enjoyed the privilege of hearing the experiences of other group members.

Wisdom comes from life experience, well digested. It's not what comes from reading great books. When it comes to understanding life, experiential learning is the only worthwhile kind; everything else is hearsay.
—Joan Erikson

We do not change as we grow older; we just become more clearly ourselves.
—Lynn Hall

Thank all participants again for attending the workshop and for sharing their stories and their trust. Remind everyone that sharing has been done in confidence and that no information shared in trust should be repeated outside the group.

Encourage participants to take time to honor their writing in the way they present it to others, even if only in a three-ring binder. Even the small effort of putting pages in a binder will help prevent the stories they have worked so hard on from getting lost.

Wish everyone well, sharing these thoughts: Adulthood is a continuing path of development. We are all still becoming. We already have survived a lot. Chances are quite good that a group of survivors like us will be able to handle whatever lies ahead. Continue to grow and learn. Seize the moments. Enjoy the adventures. Notice the details. Engage fully in the moments you share with others. Let people know who you are. Leave a legacy for future generations. Celebrate your competence, your uniqueness, your potential, and your special significance in this great family of humanity.

13. Allow time for goodbyes
As group members say goodbye, with hugs all around, remind them to pick up rosters as they leave. Encourage people to keep in touch with one other, to continue to be resources for one another. If the large group or small groups have expressed an interest in reunions, the group leader, small-group facilitators, or designated participants will take responsibility for organizing a get-together, maybe a dinner or lunch meeting, within the next two months.

APPENDIXES

A. Sample Publicity
Press Release
Fliers

B. Session Handouts
Enrollment List
Information Form
Workshop Outline
Goals and Guidelines for Group Participants
Rules for Group Leaders and Facilitators
THEME 1: *The Major Branching Points in Your Life*
Your Life Graph
Sample Life Graph
THEME 2: *Your Family*
Writing Tips
THEME 3: *The Role of Money in Your Life*
THEME 4: *Your Major Life Work or Career*
THEME 5: *Your Health and Body*
THEME 6: *Your Sexual Identity*
THEME 7: *Your Experiences with and Ideas about Death*
Where to Go from Here?
THEME 8: *Your Spiritual Life and Values*
Your Life Portfolio
Sample Life Portfolio
Abilities, Opportunities, and Responsibilities
THEME 9: *Your Goals and Aspirations*
Evaluation Form
Choosing the Title of the Story of Your Life

C. Creating New Themes

D. Adapting Workshop Schedules
Sample One-Day Program

APPENDIX A

Sample Publicity

Press Release

Date_____
For immediate release [or]
For inclusion in the [issue date] of the [publication name]

From: Name of organization
Contact: Name of contact person, telephone: 000-000-0000

AARP SPONSORS
TEN-WEEK AUTOBIOGRAPHY WORKSHOP

The Pacific Palisades Chapter of the American Association of Retired Persons (AARP) and the UCLA Center on Aging will cosponsor a ten-week workshop on guided autobiography beginning January 00, 2001, at the UCLA Extension Center in Westwood.

This workshop provides structure for anyone of any age who is interested in writing an autobiography. Each week, members of the group, under the guidance of an experienced leader, will explore a different life theme that has been influential in shaping their lives. Participants write two pages on each theme at home and bring their writing to share in a small group with others also sharing their stories.

"We start by asking participants to write down the history of branching points in their lives," says James E. Birren, Ph.D., associate director of the UCLA Center on Aging. Then in subsequent sessions, participants explore such topics as family, the role of money in one's life, one's major life work or career, health and body, and other topics that interweave to form the tapestry of a life.

Dr. Birren developed this guided autobiography technique to help would-be autobiographers find structure and meaning in the multitude of seemingly random events that compose a life.

"In five decades of studying adult development and aging," Birren says, "I have found that writing about our life experiences and sharing them with others is one of the best ways we have of giving new meaning to our present lives by understanding the past more fully."

Guided autobiography is useful to people interested in beginning an autobiography or memoir, more fully understanding the meaning of their life, or finding knowledge in the past to help them live their present and future lives in more meaningful ways. It is particularly helpful to people facing any major life transition, such as divorce, retirement, career change, parenthood, a move, or health problems.

The cost of the ten-week course is $ _____. For further information and registration, call 000-000-0000.

Flier 1

Since you are like no other being ever created since the
beginning of time, you are incomparable.
—Brenda Ueland

WRITING THE STORY OF YOUR LIFE

Would you like to participate in a guided autobiography group?

Our lives may seem to be a random and monotonous series of incidents, but they are
something more than that; each has a plot. You can learn from writing your own story and
sharing it in confidence with others who are writing theirs. This is an opportunity to explore
where you have been, where you are, and where you are going.

Who would benefit?

Men and women of all ages have benefited from the insight and personal discovery guided
autobiography provides. The process is especially beneficial for people entering or wanting to
enter a new phase of life or a new direction. Small sharing groups are especially rich when the
participants come from varied ages and backgrounds.

How is the workshop set up?

The workshop includes ten three-hour sessions. Each meeting includes instruction on
autobiography, some tools and perspectives to help inspire your writing, and time to meet in
small groups to share your writing. Each week you will be asked to write two pages on a
significant theme of your life history. We will provide priming questions to help you think
about the theme you are exploring. People who think they can't write are surprised at how
well they do because they are writing about material that means so much to them.

When and where is the workshop?

The guided autobiography workshop will meet at Smithville Presbyterian Church, Wednesday, April 00, 2001, through Wednesday, June 00, 2001. Enrollment is limited, and time will
be determined by the majority preference. Please indicate your preference:

_____ Wednesday mornings 8:30 A.M. to 10:00 A.M. in the Church Library

_____ Wednesday evenings 7:30 P.M. to 9:00 P.M. in the Multipurpose Room

The cost is $ _____ .

Name (print) _____ Phone _____

Address _____

To register, send your check and this form to Smithville Presbyterian Church,
[Street address, City, State, Zip]. For more information, call 000-000-0000.

Flier 2

[SIDE 1]

The Pacific Palisades Chapter of the AARP
and the
UCLA Center on Aging
present the

GUIDED AUTOBIOGRAPHY GROUP

Ten Monday nights, starting January 00, 2001
7:00 to 9:00 P.M.
at the Small Town Community Center
[Street address]
[City, State, Zip]
Cost $ _____

[SIDE 2]

Where have you been? Where are you now? Where are you going?
This is your chance to

- Sharpen your memories
- Write your autobiography
- Learn more about the meaning of your life
- Share your story with others

Enrollment is limited to fifteen people. Group participants will be enrolled in order of registration received. Please complete and return the registration form below with your $ _____ check made out to [Name of organization].

For more information, call 000-000-0000.

I wish to enroll in the **Guided Autobiography Group** that meets 1/00/01 to 3/00/01

Name _____ Phone _____

Address _____

City _____ State _____ Zip _____

Mail to: [Name of organization, Street address, City, State, Zip]

Flier 3

WRITING FOR YOUR LIFE

A Workshop on Guided Autobiography
9:00 A.M. to 3:30 P.M., Saturday, September 00, 2001
at the Kensington Home [Street address, City, State]

Autobiography is a powerful tool for personal and spiritual development.
Our lives may seem to be a random and monotonous series of incidents, but each has a plot. Writing a guided autobiography focused on central themes in our lives can give new meaning to our present and future lives because it helps us understand the past more fully.

Who would benefit?
This workshop is designed for clergy and church leaders interested in learning the techniques of guided autobiography in order to offer classes or workshops in their home congregations. Men and women of all ages have benefited from the insight and personal discovery guided autobiography provides. The process is especially beneficial for people seeking new direction in life. Small sharing groups are particularly rich when the participants are of varied ages and backgrounds.

How is the workshop set up?
Through lectures, guided exercises, and small-group sessions, participants will learn the basic principles of guided autobiography and leave with a format for an eight- to ten-week course.

Who will present the workshop?
James Birren, associate director, UCLA Center on Aging
Richard Myer, retired Lutheran minister
Kathryn Cochran, teacher, writer, and editor

The cost is $ _____.

Name (print)_____ Phone _____

Address _____

To register, send your check and this form to [Name of contact person], Kensington Home, [Street address, City, State, Zip]. For more information, call 000-000-0000.

APPENDIX B

Session Handouts

ENROLLMENT LIST

Please confirm or enter your name and phone number and initial the session date.

Last Name/First Name/Telephone Number	Date	Date	Date	Date	Date	Date	Date	Date	Date	Date	Date	Date
1.												
2.												
3.												
4.												
5.												
6.												
7.												
8.												
9.												
10.												
11.												
12.												
13.												
14.												
15.												
16.												
17.												
18.												
19.												
20.												
21.												
22.												
23.												
24.												
25.												

INFORMATION FORM

Name _____

Address _____

City _____ State _____ Zip _____

Phone Number w. (   ) _____ h. (   ) _____

Male ___ Female ___ Age _____ E-mail _____

Education:

Major life work:

Name(s) of spouse or friends attending with you _____

On the reverse side, please write your goals for this workshop and some interesting fact about yourself.

Workshop Outline

SESSION 1, DATE _____

Introductions
What is guided autobiography?
Goals
The importance of confidentiality
Exercises to stimulate memories
Introduce theme 1: The major branching points in your life

SESSION 2, DATE _____

Discuss problems of focus
How to draw on all the senses
Discuss goals and expectations
Introduce theme 2: Your family
Read and discuss: The major branching points in your life

SESSION 3, DATE _____

Writing tips
The power of metaphor
Introduce theme 3: The role of money in your life
Read and discuss: Your family

SESSION 4, DATE _____

Discuss concepts and elements of self-awareness
Introduce theme 4: Your major life work or career
Read and discuss: The role of money in your life

SESSION 5, DATE _____

Discuss various perspectives on human development
Introduce theme 5: Your health and body
Read and discuss: Your major life work or career

SESSION 6, DATE _____

Distinguish between writing personal history and interpreting one's life
Discuss the role of humor in guided autobiography
Introduce theme 6: Your sexual identity
Read and discuss: Your health and body

SESSION 7, DATE _____

Finding balance through confidant relationships
Introduce theme 7: Your experiences with and ideas about death
Read and discuss: Your sexual identity

SESSION 8, DATE _____

Introduce theme 8: Your spiritual life and values
Read and discuss: Your experience with and ideas about death

SESSION 9, DATE _____

Balancing your life portfolio
Introduce theme 9: Your goals and aspirations
Read and discuss: Your spiritual life and values

SESSION 10, DATE _____

Think of titles for your autobiography and its chapters
Discuss where to go from here
Hand in evaluations
Read and discuss: Your goals and aspirations
Closing comments

Goals and Guidelines for Group Participants

Goal 1: To refresh and recall the memories and events of our lives,
to organize our life histories and to share them with others
Be prepared each session to read two pages of your life story.

Goal 2: To attend all sessions
If you know in advance that you have a serious conflict and must be absent, let the workshop leader and your small-group facilitator know.

Goal 3: To complete all writing assignments
If you must miss a session, bring your two pages to the next session. Your small-group facilitator will try to make time for you to summarize what you wrote.

Goal 4: To listen actively when others are sharing
Listen attentively. You can learn from the stories of others.

Goal 5: To be supportive of others and accepting of individual differences
Avoid interpreting or analyzing what others read or say. Instead, be supportive, encouraging, and empathetic. Do not make judgmental statements about the choices other participants have made or about their feelings, beliefs, or opinions.

For example, "It must have been difficult to feel so alone"; "You showed courage to try something new when you felt so unsure." Not, "You had a classic inferiority complex."

Goal 6: To share time equally among participants
Help ensure that everyone has equal time to share his or her story. Avoid dominating the discussion, and do what you can to draw quieter members into the exchange.

Goal 7: To participate fully in writing, sharing, and discussion
What you get from the group is a reflection of what you give to it. Nevertheless, you have a right to share only what you feel comfortable sharing. If you prefer not to share part of what you have written, just skip it. Do not pressure other group members to share material they do not wish to share.

Goal 8: To limit distractions during discussion
Keep eating and other distracting noises to a minimum.

Goal 9: To respect the confidentiality of all shared information

Confidentiality is essential to trust within the group. Honor confidentiality absolutely.

Goal 10: To enjoy ourselves

Do all you can to enhance the enjoyment that comes naturally from writing and sharing your life stories.

Rules for Group Leaders and Facilitators

1. During the first session, pass out the "Goals and Guidelines for Group Participants" and read them, with elaborating comments. Encourage questions to begin group interaction and conversation.

2. Talk about the need to share time fairly.

3. Discuss the benefits of rotating the order of reading and sharing each week so that different people begin and end the sharing process.

4. When it fits and supports the flow, share incidental comments about your background so that the group feels it knows you, but don't overdo it. Above all, don't upstage other group members. Your role is to bring out the life stories of the participants, not your own.

5. Members of your group may get emotional while reading their work. Let them read through it before offering supporting comments. Tears should be treated as a normal part of life, not as some unusual event. Use humor to relax the group. Ad lib humor is great, as are appropriate humorous stories.

6. Remind participants that the questions accompanying the theme assignments needn't be answered literally. They are designed to stimulate recall of memories.

7. Tell participants they do not have to share their entire life histories. The themes gradually go to deeper, more personal areas of life, but what participants share is always their choice. Introducing difficult material too early can be uncomfortable for everyone. Explain that group members can take time to get to know one another and build trust.

8. If one participant dominates the discussion, remind the individual and the group of the importance of sharing time. Say something like, "What you have said is very interesting. I would like to hear what others have to say. Lucy, would you like to read now?" Or, "Did this trigger any memories for you, David?"

9. Some people worry about the quality of their writing. Provide gentle encouragement by saying, "We aren't all equally comfortable with writing, but we all have stories to tell. Don't worry too much about style. Just remember the events and feelings that were important to you and get them down on paper. If you focus on that instead of on style, you'll be surprised to find that you are a better writer than you thought."

10. Occasionally, members of the group will have a professional background or experience in therapy that makes them feel capable of prescribing an interpretation of life events. Remind such people that guided autobiography is not therapy, and its purpose is not to interpret other people's lives. The goal of guided autobiography is simply to help people tell life stories in everyday language. Any interpretation comes spontaneously to the individuals themselves as they integrate and write down the important experiences in their lives.

WHEN THE SMALL-GROUP FACILITATORS are also full participants in the autobiography workshop, they must wear two hats: (1) watching time and being sure that everyone shares the time fairly and that the feedback is supportive and encouraging, and (2) taking an appropriate share of time for their own reading and feedback from the group.

Theme 1: The Major Branching Points in Your Life

Branching points are the turning points in our lives—the events, experiences, or insights that significantly affected the direction or flow of our life journey. Branching points are the experiences that shape our lives in some important way. They may be big events, such as marriage, travel, a move to a new city, or retirement. Or they may be small events, such as reading a book or going on a hike. Big outcomes may have small beginnings.

Think of your life as a branching tree. Your life has many points of juncture—branches that sprout after pruning, others that atrophy for lack of nourishment. Or think of your life as a river. Where is the source? Where did branches add volume, strength, or speed? What were the impacts of storms, flood, or drought? What dams or logjams caused you to change course? What are the events that caused the turning points?

SENSITIZING QUESTIONS

These questions are designed to prime or stimulate your memories and thoughts about your life. The questions are not meant to be answered in a literal manner. Read through them and react to the ones that open windows on your past. Each life is unique, and the priming questions do not have the same value to all persons.

1.   What was the earliest branching point in your life? What happened, and why was it important? How old were you at the time?

2.   Who influenced the direction of your life in a major way? Which people were involved with you at the branching points (e.g., family, friends, teachers, doctors, lawyers, a political or religious leader, or others)?

3.   Tornadoes, fires, floods, and automobile accidents leave changed lives behind them. Were there any important happenings in your environment, either natural or societal crises, that changed the direction of your life?

4.   Were there any lucky events in your life, such as winning a lottery, getting a new job, or falling in love with the right person, that had a positive influence on the direction your life took?

5.   Were there any bad events, such as divorce, death, or illness, that influenced your life or caused it to branch?

6.   Did your ethnic, religious, or cultural background or your social or financial status have an influence on the branching points of your life? Has your background been an advantage or a disadvantage to you?

7.   Did a family change of residence or a change of school have an important impact on your life?

8. Did changing a job have lasting positive or negative effects on the flow of your life?

9. What branching points in your life were you responsible for, in contrast to branching points caused by outside events or other people?

10. Have there been any branching points in your life about which you have changed your views over time? For example, events you were angry about then and feel contented about now?

11. Do you think the flow of your life is typical of most people's lives, or is it unusual? In what ways is it unusual?

Your Life Graph

On the graph, place a dot at your age for each major event or branching point in your life. Judge the event for the way you feel about it, plus or minus. How positive or negative do you feel about the event? Connect the dots representing major events in your life to create your lifeline. Draw a vertical line for your present age, and project your lifeline into the future. How long do you expect to live, and how do you expect to feel about the years ahead?

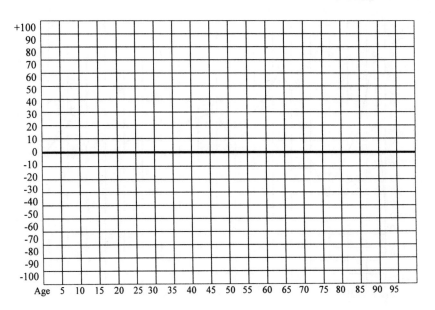

Sample Life Graph

On the graph, place a dot at your age for each major event or branching point in your life. Judge the event for the way you feel about it, plus or minus. How positive or negative do you feel about the event? Connect the dots representing major events in your life to create your lifeline. Draw a vertical line for your present age, and project your lifeline into the future. How long do you expect to live, and how do you expect to feel about the years ahead?

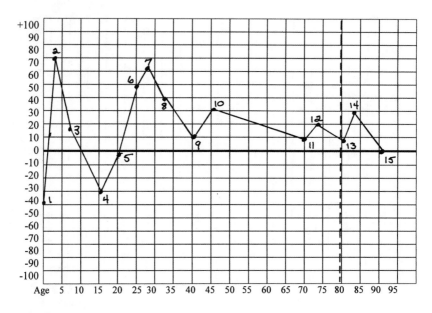

1. Birth problem (health)	6. Graduate school	11. Retirement as dean
2. Moving to rural area	7. Marriage	12. New university position
3. Starting school	8. Family	13. Retirement
4. Struggle with religion	9. Career contraction	14. Completion of books
5. Finishing junior college	10. Career expansion	15. Possible death

Theme 2: Your Family

Our family histories include both our families of origin (parents, siblings, grandparents, aunts, uncles, and cousins) and the family or families of our adult lives (spouses, children [including adopted children], grandchildren, and in-laws). Perhaps a friend or another person has been close to you and your family and has been important in your life.

What were the origins of the branches of your family? Did your family history have any impact on the directions your life took? Which family members were important in shaping your life? Some may have been important to you in positive ways and some in negative ways. Why did these family members have more impact on your life than did others?

SENSITIZING QUESTIONS

These questions are designed to prime or stimulate your memories and thoughts about your life. The questions are not meant to be answered in a literal manner. Read through them and react to the ones that open windows on your past. Each life is unique, and the priming questions do not have the same value to all persons.

1. Who held the power in your family and made the major decisions? How do you know?
2. Which family members have you felt closest to, and which ones felt most distant? Why? Were or are any family members your models in life?
3. Did you like your family and feel supported and loved?
4. Were there any family members you were afraid of?
5. What were the rules in your family about eating, cleaning up, dressing, and so forth? When you sat down to dinner, where did you sit?
6. Did your family have any hero figures who had stories told about them?
7. Did your family have any odd figures who were ridiculed, such as a miser or a spendthrift, a noisy or talkative person or a silent one?
8. What were the strengths and weaknesses in your family? How did they affect you?
9. Were there any events that made your family stronger or tore it apart?
10. What is the history of your family? What were its origins, and who were its major figures?
11. Did your family have a philosophy about life that was discussed and that you were expected to adopt? What were the "shoulds" and "oughts" in your family? What favorite sayings illustrate your family's philosophy of life?
12. Is there anything about your family that seems unusual to you?

Writing Tips

1. Use active, not passive verbs.
This keeps the action and the reader's attention moving forward.

> *"Rick threw the ball into left field."*

> *Not, "The ball was thrown into left field by Rick."*

2. Use all the senses.

> *"The thunder boomed through the night, and static electricity in the air made the hair on our forearms stand up straight."*

> *"In Grandma's kitchen the sweet smell of fresh strawberries combined with the lingering aroma of bacon grease and coffee from breakfast."*

3. Give each writing assignment all the best stuff you have.
When you go back to the well, miraculously, there is always more to work with, so there's no need to save material for later.

4. Show, don't tell.
Paint a picture with words.

> *"Uncle Abraham was so honest he would walk five miles to return the correct change to a customer."*

> *Not, "Uncle Abraham was honest."*

5. Use concrete detail and avoid abstractions.
The facts won't change over time. Your interpretations might.

> *"Uncle Ed, Ma, Sissy and my brother Joe were all in the Model A, already pointed west. Dad and I brought out the last box, Grandma's china wrapped in rags and towels so [it] wouldn't break on the way to California. Ma wanted to hold the dishes on her own lap. So Dad handed them to her, turned and spit in the dust and climbed into the driver's seat."*

> *Not, "Like hundreds of other families, we moved to California during the Great Depression."*

6. Write straight to the emotional core of things.

You are writing about your childhood, the time when you found everything so intensely interesting and felt things so deeply. You are writing about your adolescence with all its roller coaster emotions, idealism, and realizations, and about your continuing development as an adult. Don't be too distant. Write with care and truth and with empathy and understanding for that child, that young person, and the person you are now. Try to understand what he or she was feeling. Help others to learn from that child's experience, from the experience of a human being trying to make sense of life.

Exploring your life and understanding the child that you were will give you insight and compassion. You will see the details in a different light. You may notice things you hadn't noticed before. And when you share, you will turn on a light for others so they can see the significance of their own lives more clearly.

Theme 3: The Role of Money in Your Life

Money is an important factor in most lives and can have both obvious and subtle influences on the way we live. Money can touch many aspects of our lives, including family life, where we live, education, health, relationships with others, and self-esteem. The history of how we have dealt with money and our ideas about money are important aspects of our life stories. Our attitudes toward money have been shaped by many influences, both positive and negative.

SENSITIZING QUESTIONS

These questions are designed to prime or stimulate your memories and thoughts about your life. The questions are not meant to be answered in a literal manner. Read through them and react to the ones that open windows on your past. Each life is unique, and the priming questions do not have the same value to all persons.

1. What role did money play in your family? Was money scarce or plentiful? How did your family's financial situation compare with that of other people you knew? Did your family think of itself as being well-off or poor?
2. What were you taught about money? Who gave you most of your ideas about money?
3. Did money have any relationship to affection and love in your family?
4. What was the first time you earned any money? How did it influence your later ideas?
5. In your life, how important has it been to make money?
6. How much do you think about money or worry about it?
7. What have been your greatest successes with money? Your worst mistakes? Are you a good or poor manager of money?
8. Have you ever had to borrow money? How did you feel about it? Have other people helped you when you needed money?
9. Does money have any relation to your self-regard or self-esteem?
10. Do you regard yourself as generous or stingy? Do you give money away? How do you feel about it? Were there any spendthrifts or misers in your family?
11. What has money come to mean to you—power, position, comfort, security, or something else?

Theme 4: Your Major Life Work or Career

Our life work includes the activities that have occupied most of our time, energy, or concerns. It can take many forms. The history of our life work may include work as a parent, spouse, or homemaker. It can be the history of a career or lifetime job. Also, it can be a lifetime of service in religion, community work, or politics. Some people devote their lives to art or literature. We may have several careers or life work activities in sequence or at the same time. What has been the pattern or the sequence of your life work?

SENSITIZING QUESTIONS

These questions are designed to prime or stimulate your memories and thoughts about your life. The questions are not meant to be answered in a literal manner. Read through them and react to the ones that open windows on your past. Each life is unique, and the priming questions do not have the same value to all persons.

1. How did you get into your major life work? Did you seem destined to follow it, or did you stumble into it? Did other persons urge you to pursue this work, or was chance a factor? Did any childhood interests or experiences influence your path?
2. When did you develop the goals of your life? How much choice did you have?
3. What events or persons influenced your path?
4. Were family models important in the life work you chose? Who influenced you the most?
5. What role did being a man or woman play in your choices about your life work?
6. Has your life work been one continuous path, or have there been changes and discontinuities? Have there been peaks and valleys?
7. Were you provided many options, or did you have only one or two prospects?
8. Are you satisfied with your life work? Is there anything you would like to change? What personal strengths or weaknesses have you brought to your life work?
9. If you have had more than one life work, which has been most important to you?
10. What have you liked most and least about your life work?
11. How did the place where you grew up and the times in which you lived influence your choices and the way in which you think about your life work?
12. If you were to live your life again, would you choose the same or a different life work?
13. On the basis of your experience, what would you say about work to a young person just starting out in adult life?

Theme 5: Your Health and Body

Health is an important influence in shaping our lives. Acute or chronic illnesses, whether experienced by ourselves or by another person in our lives, can lead to major changes in the way we live. Our views of our health and body have many aspects, including both the history of our own health and physical characteristics and our feelings about them. In part, our views involve comparisons with other persons—are we healthy or unhealthy, strong or weak, coordinated or clumsy, attractive or unattractive, compared with others? What is the history of your health and body?

SENSITIZING QUESTIONS

These questions are designed to prime or stimulate your memories and thoughts about your life. The questions are not meant to be answered in a literal manner. Read through them and react to the ones that open windows on your past. Each life is unique, and the priming questions do not have the same value to all persons.

1. How was your health when you were a baby, child, and adult? Have any serious illnesses or accidents changed the way you lived? In what ways?
2. What health problems have you experienced over the course of your life? How did they influence you?
3. Were you considered a well child or a sickly child? Did it make any difference to you?
4. Were you fast- or slow-developing as a child? Were you ahead of or behind your peers in growth and development as an adolescent? How did this affect your image of yourself?
5. How would you describe yourself as a child, adolescent, or adult? Were you short or tall, thin or fat, poised or awkward? As a male or female, would you regard yourself as attractive or unattractive?
6. How has your body reacted to sports and exercise?
7. How has your body reacted to stress? Has this changed during your life? What signals in your body indicate that you are under stress? Have you been exposed to high stress? If so, how have you responded to it?
8. What have you done during your life to help or hurt your health?
9. What aspects or parts of your body do you like best or least? If you could change your body in any way, how would you like it to be different?
10. What have you done to alter or improve your health and body during your life?

Theme 6: Your Sexual Identity

Our ideas about what it means to be a woman or a man evolve, and they come from many sources, such as family members, friends, reading, and our experiences in life. The history of our sexual development, including our identities as boys or girls, men or women, is an important aspect of our personal histories. Our concepts of appropriate sex-role behavior may change over the course of life.

SENSITIZING QUESTIONS

These questions are designed to prime or stimulate your memories and thoughts about your life. The questions are not meant to be answered in a literal manner. Read through them and react to the ones that open windows on your past. Each life is unique, and the priming questions do not have the same value to all persons.

1. When did you first realize that you were a girl or a boy and that boys and girls were different? How did you feel about it?
2. What did your family tell you about being a boy or girl and how you should behave? Did your family have different rules for boys' and girls' behavior?
3. What kind of clothes did you wear when you were a child? What kinds of toys and games did you play? Were any kinds of games forbidden?
4. What did your parents, teachers, and others tell you about what good girls and boys did and did not do? What were your parents' views about your sexuality?
5. Were you ever called a sissy, a tomboy, or a 'fraidy cat? Did you ever wish you were of the opposite sex?
6. When and where did you get your education about sex or the facts of life? What were your primary sources of information—a family member, school friends, reading, movies, or religion?
7. How have your ideas about the ideal man or the ideal woman developed? How would you characterize yourself as a man or a woman?
8. Did you have any childhood sweethearts? What were your early sexual experiences?
9. Have you had any traumatic sexual experiences? Are there any sexual experiences you regret?
10. Have your ideas about appropriate sexual behavior changed? What are your ideas about the ideal relationships between men and women?
11. Do you feel contemporary ideas about men, women, and sexuality have changed? If so, how do you relate to the new ideas?
12. Have your sexual experiences and identity been influenced by changes with age, health, retirement, or bereavement?

Theme 7: Your Experiences with and Ideas about Death

Death can affect our lives in many ways. As children, we may have experienced the loss of a pet. Later, we may have lost parents, grandparents, a spouse, child, brother, sister, or a close friend. The death of a national hero may have affected us profoundly. The circumstances of deaths and our age at the time they occurred can have long-lasting influences. How have your experiences with death affected your life and your personal philosophy?

SENSITIZING QUESTIONS

These questions are designed to prime or stimulate your memories and thoughts about your life. The questions are not meant to be answered in a literal manner. Read through them and react to the ones that open windows on your past. Each life is unique, and the priming questions do not have the same value to all persons.

1. What did you feel about death as a child? Did you lose an animal that was like a member of the family? What did you think when your pet died?
2. How was death talked about and treated in your family? Did it frighten you?
3. How were family funerals and memorial services held? When did you go to your first funeral? What did you think about it, and how did you react?
4. Did any wartime deaths affect you? If so, what were their circumstances?
5. Have you ever been responsible for anyone's death? How did you feel about it then and now?
6. Have you had any close calls with death, such as an illness or accident?
7. Do any deceased persons, such as a parent, spouse, or friend, continue to have an effect on your life?
8. Have you been closely involved with anyone's death? How have you grieved? How do you feel about it—guilty, resentful, angry, or peaceful? Were some deaths welcomed?
9. What was the most significant death you experienced? How did it change your life?
10. Did the death of some well-known person (e.g., Gandhi, John or Robert Kennedy, or Martin Luther King, Jr.) have an effect on you?
11. How have your ideas about death evolved? What kind of death would you like to have? Is death a friend for you, or is it to be fought, dreaded, or accepted?
12. If you could talk with someone who has died, what would you say or ask?

Where to Go from Here?

As we discussed at the beginning of this workshop, guided autobiography is really a kind of fishing expedition. By now you have done a lot of writing and know that each two-page piece you have written could be expanded into a book. You have learned a great deal about yourself and your colleagues. What now? Subsequent courses? Starting a group of your own? Publishing? Preparing a scrapbook for family? A video? Reunions with this group?

In the final session we will take time to discuss where to go from here. Please take some time before our next session to write down on this page your questions, goals, and ideas so that I can be as prepared as possible to respond to your needs. Others in this group will have ideas, too. Let's see how we can help each other continue to grow.

Please hand in this information at the beginning of the next session.

Theme 8: Your Spiritual Life and Values

Our spiritual histories include experiences with people, nature, and religion that have contributed to the development of our philosophies of life and that part of us that cannot be defined in purely physical terms. The history of our spiritual lives and values need not be confined to experiences in church or in organized religion, although for some persons those experiences may play an important part. What is the history of your quest for values, truth, and meaning in life? What people, experiences, readings, and inspirations have guided you in your spiritual journey?

SENSITIZING QUESTIONS

These questions are designed to prime or stimulate your memories and thoughts about your life. The questions are not meant to be answered in a literal manner. Read through them and react to the ones that open windows on your past. Each life is unique, and the priming questions do not have the same value to all persons.

1. Do you remember having a spiritual experience when you were growing up that gave you a feeling of belonging and being special in the universe or a feeling of rejection and loneliness? What was it like?
2. As a child, what kind of instruction and ideas were you given of a spiritual, religious, or philosophical nature? Did your family discuss such things?
3. Did you have an early image of God? Where did it come from? What was it like?
4. Were you ever challenged to take a stand on religion, state your faith, or defend your values?
5. Did your family or outside influences have a greater impact on shaping your values and beliefs? Which persons had the most influence on your ideas?
6. When you first left home for a long time, did that change your outlook on life, values, or personal philosophy?
7. What books made an impression on you, spiritually or morally?
8. What have been your relationships with organized religion? How important have they been in your outlook and the way you have lived your life? Did you ever break with a church you belonged to? If so, how did the break evolve?
9. Did you ever have a spiritual or religious experience that had an important impact on the way you lived your life? Did you ever have any experiences of deep faith, conviction, or peace?
10. What friends, mentors, or role models have helped you on your spiritual path?
11. How would you describe your spiritual quest at this time? What have you learned, and what are you struggling to understand?

Your Life Portfolio

Just as a diversified portfolio of financial investments provides balance and strength in an unpredictable world, a balanced investment of the time, energy, and concern we devote to various aspects of our life portfolio makes us more resilient. Your life portfolio merits periodic evaluation to see whether the way you have been distributing your time and energy still makes sense. This graph is designed to give you a picture of how you have been investing your life energy and encourages you to think about how you want to divide those energies in the future.

On a piece of paper, make two columns. Using a pencil so you can erase if you want to, list the percentage of time and energy you devote to each of the ten activities listed in the chart below. One column should represent the present, the other your goals for the future. Each column should add up to 100 percent.

Now chart the percentages with circles on the graph and connect the circles. Use a solid line for the present and a dashed line for the future.

When you have finished, share your goals with someone else who has completed the exercise. What specific changes will you have to make to achieve your goals? What steps have to be taken? Can you pin each step to a time frame?

A goal such as "I'm going to make two phone calls a week to let friends know I am thinking of them" is more likely to induce real change than a vague goal such as "I'm going to spend more time with friends."

PERCENTAGE OF TIME AND ENERGY INVESTED

	0	20	40	60	80	100
Family						
Friends						
Health and Body						
Homemaking						
Career and work						
Money						
Education						
Leisure/hobbies						
Religion						
Public Service						

Sample Life Portfolio

Just as a diversified portfolio of financial investments provides balance and strength in an unpredictable world, a balanced investment of the time, energy, and concern we devote to various aspects of our life portfolio makes us more resilient. Your life portfolio merits periodic evaluation to see whether the way you have been distributing your time and energy still makes sense. This graph is designed to give you a picture of how you have been investing your life energy and encourages you to think about how you want to divide those energies in the future.

On a piece of paper, make two columns. Using a pencil so you can erase if you want to, list the percentage of time and energy you devote to each of the ten activities listed in the chart below. One column should represent the present, the other your goals for the future. Each column should add up to 100 percent.

Now chart the percentages with circles on the graph and connect the circles. Use a solid line for the present and a dashed line for the future.

When you have finished, share your goals with someone else who has completed the exercise. What specific changes will you have to make to achieve your goals? What steps have to be taken? Can you pin each step to a time frame?

A goal such as "I'm going to make two phone calls a week to let friends know I am thinking of them" is more likely to induce real change than a vague goal such as "I'm going to spend more time with friends."

PERCENTAGE OF TIME AND ENERGY INVESTED

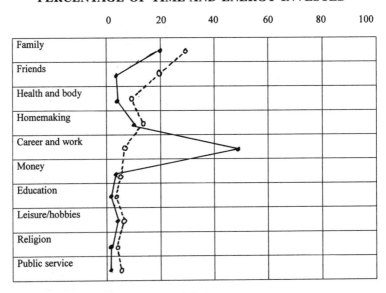

Abilities, Opportunities, and Responsibilities

As we review our life portfolios and evaluate where we want to put our energies, we might draw some inspiration from some statements about life's responsibilities by James Birren.

1. I should honor my children and all children and foster their growth. May I remain close to my children, but not hover over them and stunt their maturity.

2. I should avoid becoming bitter if overlooked by the passing young and events of time. May the acids of life not erode my spirit. I should not blame or rage against others for their inability to control the impossible.

3. I should continue to seek information and learning and avoid dogmatic positions and postures. May I be a source of experience for solving or moderating the problems of life.

4. I should use the experience of my years for attaining fairness and justice for others.

5. I should foster my physical and mental health. Should I have poor health, I should cushion its impact so that it does not weigh unduly upon others. I should refrain from seeking an unreasonable share of resources and placing a disproportionate load upon others.

6. I should manage prudently and with affection my relationships with others and initiate the expressions of caring and love for others. May I manage the passage of possessions with fairness and avoid manipulating them to gain attention or to cause others to vie for material gain.

7. I should continue to weed the garden of my life, remove yesterday's flowers and dead branches and foster new growth.

8. I should prepare others and myself for my death. May I promote my passing with poise, dignity, and peace. I should consider making provisions for the use by others of my body parts.

9. I should leave the land and its people better than I found them. May I have planted seeds that will bloom for others in springs I will not see.

Theme 9: Your Goals and Aspirations

Our goals and aspirations are an important part of our life stories. An account of how we grew up and lived our life includes the goals we have had and the things we have been striving for. Our goals and aspirations form an integral part of the fabric of our lives. For some persons, goals may remain the same throughout life, but this is not necessarily true for everyone. Experience may have taught us that we should change our goals or trade in our aspirations for new ones that better fit with the realities of our lives or our changing values. What have you been working to attain or achieve in your life, and what kind of person have you tried to be?

SENSITIZING QUESTIONS

These questions are designed to prime or stimulate your memories and thoughts about your life. The questions are not meant to be answered in a literal manner. Read through them and react to the ones that open windows on your past. Each life is unique, and the priming questions do not have the same value to all persons.

1. When you were a child, whom did you want to be like, or what kind of person did you want to become when you grew up? Did your role models change during adolescence? In what way?
2. Where did you find your models—in the family, movies, or other sources?
3. Which characteristics of your ideal self or ideal model were most important to you—accomplishments, athletic ability, appearance, money, reputation, creativity, philosophy, religion, or something else?
4. In your school years, what were your goals? What did you want to accomplish?
5. How important were your teachers and education in shaping your goals? Did they lead to changes in your goals and your ideas about what you wanted to achieve in your life?
6. Have you changed your goals during your life? How? What experiences or major events influenced the changes?
7. What do you think have been the most important achievements of your life? Is there anything you feel so strongly about that you would sacrifice almost everything for it?
8. Which persons have had the most influence on what you wanted to achieve?
9. Did you ever have a period when you felt your life was meaningless?
10. Looking back over your life, would you now pursue different goals? What would they be?
11. What aspirations do you have now, and what goals do you have for your future?
12. What legacy would you like to create that would be a symbol of how you led your life? If you wrote a book about your life, what would its title be?

Evaluation Form

Workshop leader _____

Workshop location _____

Date _____

Part I. Circle your rating of the following guided autobiography workshop elements from 1 to 7, with 1 being poor and 7 being excellent.

Workshop Leader	Poor						Excellent
Knowledge	1	2	3	4	5	6	7
Enthusiasm for the subject	1	2	3	4	5	6	7
Preparedness	1	2	3	4	5	6	7
Small-Group Facilitator							
Skill in managing discussions	1	2	3	4	5	6	7
Background knowledge	1	2	3	4	5	6	7
Preparedness	1	2	3	4	5	6	7
The Workshop							
Evaluation of the total experience	1	2	3	4	5	6	7
Extent to which the course met your expectations	1	2	3	4	5	6	7

Part II.

1. What were the most and least satisfactory features about the large-group sessions?

    a. Most _____

    _____

    b. Least _____

    _____

2. What were the most and least satisfactory features of the small-group sessions?

   c. Most _____

   _____

   d. Least _____

   _____

3. What recommendations would you make to improve the program? _____

   _____

   _____

   _____

Part III. Rate the following features by placing an X in the appropriate box.

	Very Satisfactory	**Satisfactory**	**Not Satisfactory**
1. Day and Time			
2. Parking			
3. Refreshments			
4. Handouts			
5. Other_____			

Choosing the Title of the Story of Your Life

If you think of your autobiography as a story of life, take time to think about a provocative title for your story. What is the central theme of your life story? If you were publishing your autobiography, what would the title be?

The following examples are provided to stimulate your thoughts about the core themes of your life.

Edward Blishen, *Sorry, Dad*
Charles L. Blockson, *Damn Rare: The Memoirs of an African American Bibliophile*
David Daiches, *Two Worlds: An Edinburgh Jewish Childhood*
M. K. Gandhi, *The Story of My Experiments with Truth*
H. Peter Kriendler, *Everyday Was New Year's Eve: Memoirs of a Saloon Keeper*
Ibbie Ledford, *Hill Country Cookin' and Memoirs*
Terry O'Sullivan, *Did I Miss Anything? Memoirs of a Soap Opera Star*
Anwar el-Sadat, *In Search of an Identity*
Pat Schroeder, *Twenty-four Years of House Work and the Place Is Still a Mess*
Barbara Probst Solomon, *Arriving Where We Started*

Here are some other possibilities for autobiography titles.

The Story of My Life: I Had to Do It Alone
The Story of My Life: Life Was Tough, but I Was Tougher
The Story of My Life: People Are the Most
The Story of My Life: Taking Charge

On the back of this paper, write down as many phrases as you can think of that might describe your life. Some examples:

Work, Work, Nothing but Work
Flying High: Memoirs of a Pilot
Sole Food: Memoirs of a Country Walker
Hey, Mom! Where's the . . . ?
I Did All That, and More

This is a brainstorming session. Write down every idea, then pick the three you like best and create three titles. Write them below:

1. _____

2. _____

3. _____

Which one seems best? Why?

Creating New Themes

A guided autobiography workshop can be organized in a variety of ways. We encourage leaders to adapt the number and subjects of life themes to the needs and interests of a particular group. Groups with common goals or backgrounds, such as university alumni, veterans, church members, housing project neighbors, or AARP chapter members, may gain access to their memories through specially created themes. When creating new themes, keep the following points in mind.

1. The stage should be set with an opening paragraph.

A theme should open with a short paragraph that sets the stage for recollections and for the priming or sensitizing questions that follow. For example, if one were creating a guided autobiography group for college alumni, the following stage-setting opening might be suitable.

Your College Life

Being in college can bring with it many changes as we make new friends, attend classes, and perhaps adjust to living for the first time apart from our families. New ideas may arise, and we may learn more about ourselves as we see and talk to others. What were your experiences with being in college? Think about the questions below and write about your education and growing up.

A similar introductory paragraph might prepare veterans groups for the flood of memories the priming questions bring up.

Your War Experiences

Being in military service and serving in wartime conditions can totally change a person's life. Fear, uncertainty, issues of patriotism, loyalty to comrades, the threat of death, and possibly horrific battlefield experiences, as well as separation from home and family, can powerfully influence the directions of our lives. Wartime experiences vary with the countries and regions of service, the branch of service, the men and women with whom the experience is shared, and other chance events. What was your experience in the military? Think about the questions below and write about the history of your military experiences and their effect on your life.

2. Most themes can trigger positive or negative recollections.

Virtually any theme you develop can have positive or negative associations for group participants, depending on the individuals' experiences. Word your introductory paragraph and the priming questions carefully to allow room for both pleasant and unpleasant recollections on the same topic. For example, different college alumni may remember the same professor with fondness or disdain. Priming questions should allow for either response. For example, you might ask, "When you were in school, who was the teacher you admired the most? Why?"; "Whom did you dislike the most? Why?"

For veterans, similar two-sided questions invite open and honest responses. Questions might include, for example, "Which senior officer did you respect the most? Why?"; "Which senior officer did you respect the least? Why?"

Further priming questions can be developed using positive and negative approaches to different aspects of the common experiences: "When you were in college, what aspect of college life did you like the most? Why?"; "What aspect of college life did you dislike the most? Why?"

Using positive and negative questions encourages autobiography participants to reflect on the many sides of life's experiences and tends to legitimatize their expressions of strong negative or positive feelings. For example, in the context of church groups the priming questions might include, "What was the most meaningful or important religious experience you ever had? Describe it." And the alternative, "What was the most unsettling or unpleasant religious experience you ever had? Describe it."

3. A common experience may have unequal significance for group participants.

Starting school may produce vivid memories for one person and no memories for another. The Great Depression of the 1930s had a strong impact on many lives, but some were untouched. A question might be written, "Did the Depression of the 1930s have any impact on your growing up?" Or, "Did the Vietnam War period have an impact on the way you grew up?" The point is that priming questions should be open questions that stimulate the flow of memories without encouraging stereotypes or communicating to participants that any particular answers or feelings are expected.

4. Seemingly insignificant subjects can lead by association to themes that are central to an individual's personal history.

Questions about some seemingly inconsequential aspect of life—the role of food in your life, for example—can lead to many related issues including family life, money, and health. Remembering a favorite toy may lead into issues of sibling rivalry or memories of a favorite relative who gave the toy or a picture of economic conditions in the family. Using the relatively simple themes of food and toys can create memory paths to important family relationships and fulfilled and unfulfilled aspirations in life. In the structure of a life story, big and little events all play roles and any number of topics can be used to prime the memories of the participants in autobiography groups.

5. Questions should not make participants feel any bias about the way they should think or feel about the past.

Guided autobiography is designed to help people recall and organize their life stories. The questions should support this goal and not solicit interpretation or evaluation. In writing about the facts and events of their histories, people may come to some spontaneous interpretive insights of their own, but that is not a job appropriate for the leader or for other members of the group. The leader's strategy should be to prime memories and aid in their organization, leaving the evaluations of events and people to the persons who experienced them.

One retired man in an autobiography group said, "I left research to go into university administration. Had I stayed with my research, I might have won a Nobel Prize." To the others in the group it seemed as though he had had a distinguished and enviable career. He was less certain about how to evaluate his life.

A woman who had just turned forty-five said, "I am forty-five, not married, no children, and I wonder if my career has been worth it." To others it seemed she was miles ahead in a career that was not selfishly oriented but served others, as well as providing her with a high standard of living.

The seemingly big and little features of life evoke different evaluations, and all individuals may change their personal evaluation of life events as they revisit the path that brought them to where they are.

Adapting Workshop Schedules

Guided autobiography workshop leaders may be asked to adapt the materials for shorter sessions ranging from an hour and a half to a two- or three-day weekend retreat. Such requests arise from many sources, including community organizations, religious groups, and professional organizations whose members serve older adults or other specific groups. Participants in the workshops may be interested in autobiography for themselves or for the members of the constituencies they serve.

In all instances, the workshops serve multiple purposes. The participants should leave the workshop with a perspective that encourages them to seek further information. In these abbreviated workshops, the leader's goals should be as follows:

1. To provide a limited introduction to the concepts and benefits of guided autobiography, emphasizing that this cannot replace the full ten-session experience
2. To use exercises to give participants limited exposure to group processes as a tool for stimulating the recollection of old memories
3. To introduce examples of themes and encourage audience interaction, which the leader uses to promote exchange of memories and life stories
4. To describe the sequence of topics from general to more personal to more future-oriented subjects that has proven useful in the ten-session workshop
5. To provide a brief reading list of relevant books and articles, as well as access to this manual, for more detailed information

We include here a sample program for a one-day workshop. It can be adapted for shorter sessions by eliminating some of the theme work between the introduction and conclusion. For longer, weekend workshops, include more of the theme work presented in this manual; allow time for participants to write about memories primed by the theme sheets and to read their one or two pages in groups of three. Even if you have only an hour, be sure to include sharing time about branching points or childhood memories about families or food, for example, so that participants begin to experience the power of sharing their stories with others.

Sample One-Day Program

8:30–9:00 A.M. REGISTRATION

Set up a table for display of books and literature related to autobiography.

9:00–9:45 A.M. INTRODUCTION TO GUIDED AUTOBIOGRAPHY

1. Describe the purpose and process of guided autobiography.
2. Emphasize the importance of writing *and* sharing life stories.
3. List reasons why people might want to do autobiography (from Session 1).
4. Discuss the importance of confidentiality and the role of confidant relationships in adapting to situations throughout life.
5. Ask participants to take fifteen minutes (five minutes each) to share in groups of three about a childhood memory related to food or family meals.
6. In the large group, ask for feedback about what memories other people's stories triggered and whether participants now feel warmer toward people with whom they have shared a small piece of their history.

9:45–10:30 A.M. BRANCHING POINTS IN LIFE

1. Introduce theme 1: the major branching points in your life. Share one or two major branching points from your own life and draw a few examples from workshop participants to prime the memories of others.
2. Hand out the theme sheet and go over the priming questions, noting that they do not need to be answered literally.
3. Ask the participants to share their major branching points in groups of three for fifteen minutes, five minutes each.

10:30–10:45 A.M. COFFEE BREAK

10:45–11:15 A.M. SMALL-GROUP DYNAMICS

1. Discuss group process and the role of small-group facilitators in a full ten-week workshop. Emphasize the following points: feedback in small groups should be affirming

and nonjudgmental, and interpretation of life events must come from the individual who is writing, not from others in the group.

2. Discuss problems that can come up in small-group dynamics and strategies for trouble-shooting.

3. Tell the group that the process of writing and sharing usually leads participants to realize that everyone has had an interesting life with direction and meaning and that we are all capable survivors!

11:15 A.M.–12:15 P.M. YOUR FAMILY

1. Point out that the sharing session on branching points just started the process of remembering and organizing the history of branching points. In a full workshop, participants would have a week to think about it and would write two pages to share in their small groups. In the group, hearing the stories of other participants then stimulates even more memories for the listeners. The process can lead to rich, rewarding, and quite fully developed life histories.

2. Introduce the second theme, your family, by sharing a few memories or characteristics of your own family. Draw a few examples from volunteers among the participants.

3. Hand out the theme sheets and go over the priming questions, giving examples where appropriate.

4. Ask participants to share in groups of three for a total of fifteen minutes.

5. Before the lunch break, ask participants whether they have any questions about the content or process of the morning sessions. Suggest that, over lunch, they continue sharing memories that may have been stimulated by themes 1 and 2. If time permits, a walk and talk with other participants after lunch may stimulate even more memories.

12:15–1:15 P.M. LUNCH

1:15–2:45 P.M. YOUR LIFE WORK OR CAREER

1. Point out that our life work may be the place where we invested most of our time and energy or interest. This might include raising children, running a household, a career outside the home, public service, volunteer work, or religious work.

2. Hand out the theme sheets and go over the priming questions, giving examples from your life and drawing examples from participants.

3. Now that participants are accustomed to sharing, allow thirty minutes of sharing in groups of three, ten minutes per participant.

2:45–3:00 P.M. COFFEE BREAK

3:00–4:00 P.M. CONCLUSION

1. Describe the remaining themes used in a full guided autobiography workshop. Describe how themes might be adapted for special group needs and how new themes can be developed for specialized groups.
2. Discuss some of the available literature on autobiography and reminiscence.
3. Hand out workshop evaluation forms. While the audience is filling out the forms, ask for questions from the floor.
4. Conclude with any of the appropriate quotations from this manual, leaving a sense that autobiography is an exciting enterprise with many worthy and rewarding applications.

Annotated Reading List

Birren, J. E., and Deutchman, D. E. 1991. *Guiding autobiography groups for older adults.* Baltimore: Johns Hopkins University Press.
   A plan for conducting groups to help people recall, organize, and tell their life stories.

Birren, J. E., and Feldman, L. 1997. *Where to go from here.* New York: Simon & Schuster.
   A practical guide to reviewing the past and exploring the future in the second half of life.

Bridges, W. 1980. *Making sense of life's changes.* Reading, Mass.: Addison-Wesley.
   A discussion of how transitions bring opportunity and turmoil, illustrated by some successful transitions that help us recognize and seize new opportunities.

Burnside, I. (ed.). 1986. *Working with the elderly: group process and techniques,* 2d ed. Boston: Jones & Bartlett.
   Many approaches to group work with the elderly, including reminiscence, described by authors from different professional orientations.

Coleman, P. G. 1986. *Ageing and reminiscence processes.* New York: John Wiley.
   An account of reminiscence as a tool for studying late-life adjustments and the role of memories.

Egan, S. 1984. *Patterns of experience in autobiography.* Chapel Hill: University of North Carolina Press.
   An analysis of autobiography from the point of view of literature and the use of myth and fiction in life stories.

Leibovits, M., and Solomon, L. 1993. *Legacies.* New York: HarperCollins.
   Life stories of humor, courage, resilience, and love by writers sixty and older.

Rainer, T. 1998 *Your life as story.* New York: Jeremy Tarcher & Putnam.
   Guidance on how to convert your life story into art, by an author with a background in both the literary and entertainment industries.

Reker, G. T., and Chamberlain, K. (eds.). 2000. *Exploring existential meaning.* Thousand Oaks, Calif.: Sage Publications.

A description of the contemporary search for meaning in life and the applications of various approaches to improving personal adjustment, by a variety of authors.

Runyan, W. M. 1982. *Life histories and psychobiography.* New York: Oxford University Press.

A review of approaches to the understanding of individual lives from the vantage points of the social sciences and humanities.

Wakefield, D. 1990. *The story of your life: writing a spiritual autobiography.* Boston: Beacon Press.

A journalist's account of how to write about and share our most meaningful experiences and, in doing so, to see our lives in a new light.

Index

James E. Birren, Ph.D., has been working with autobiography groups for more than twenty-five years. He has conducted numerous workshops on his approach across the United States and abroad. Currently, he is associate director of the University of California, Los Angeles, Center on Aging and adjunct professor in the UCLA Department of Psychiatry and Biobehavioral Sciences. He is professor emeritus of gerontology and psychology at the University of Southern California. Dr. Birren has received numerous awards for his research. He has published extensively about aging and has more than 250 publications in academic journals and books. In 1996 he edited the *Encyclopedia of Gerontology* (Academic Press), and in 1997 he published with Linda Feldman a book on autobiography, *Where to Go From Here* (Simon & Schuster).

Kathryn N. Cochran is a writer, editor, and teacher. She holds a master's degree in journalism from the University of Missouri, Columbia. Ms. Cochran has lived on three continents and written on topics ranging from basic science and engineering to the arts and architecture. She has a particular interest in human development and cross-cultural communication. Ms. Cochran met Jim Birren in 1985 when he was dean of the USC School of Gerontology and she was an editor on the USC alumni magazine. She took his autobiography class to help her father write his memoirs. Since then she has led guided autobiography workshops as well as workshops on writing and creativity.